T0291597

Download Your Included Ebook Today!

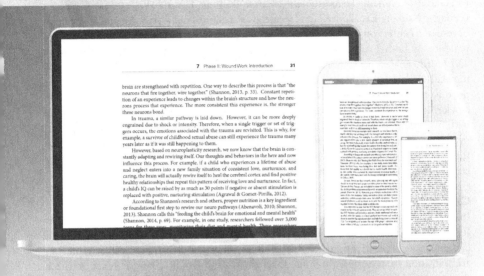

Your print purchase of *Grant Writing Handbook for Nurses and Health Professionals*, 3e, **includes an ebook download** to the device of your choice—increasing accessibility, portability, and searchability!

Download your ebook today at:
http://spubonline.com/granthbk
and enter the access code below:

1Y050DY70

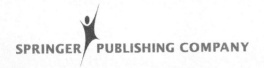

SPRINGER PUBLISHING COMPANY

BT

Barbara J. Holtzclaw, PhD, RN, FAAN, is associate dean for research and professor, Earl and Fran Ziegler College of Nursing, University of Oklahoma Health Sciences Center, Oklahoma City, Oklahoma. She also serves as doctoral faculty and associate director, Geriatric Nursing Translational Research Training, Donald W. Reynolds Center of Geriatric Nursing Excellence. Dr. Holtzclaw is a clinical nurse scientist whose program of research centers on thermoregulatory responses to illness and treatment in vulnerable patients. As both a successful grant recipient and a consultant-mentor to other nurse and health-related professionals, she is particularly well qualified to teach grant writing skills to nursing PhD students and faculty through workshops wherein she uses the third edition (2018) of *Grant Writing Handbook for Nurses and Other Health Professionals* as a key instrument. Her research funding includes four major federally funded projects, with two R01 grants to study febrile symptoms in cancer and HIV, which has supported over 50 publications on the topics of fever, shivering, hypothermia, and management of thermoregulatory responses. She is best known for translational studies in which basic science concepts are used to develop clinical nursing interventions.

Carole Kenner, PhD, RN, FAAN, FNAP, ANEF, is the Carol Kuser Loser Dean/ Professor at the School of Nursing, Health, and Exercise Science at The College of New Jersey, Ewing, New Jersey. She is also the chief executive officer and founding president of the Council of International Neonatal Nurses, Inc. (COINN). Her research interests are transition from hospital to home for neonates and families, clinical genetics within the context of family support, fetal alcohol prevention, and childhood obesity. She has successfully written National Institutes of Health, Centers for Disease Control and Prevention, Health Resources and Services Administration, corporate, and foundation grants. Dr. Kenner has authored over 100 journal articles and edited 30 textbooks. She is the recipient of numerous awards, including the Sigma Theta Tau International, Inc., Audrey Hepburn Award for her international work to support children

Marlene Walden, PhD, APRN, NNP-BC, CCNS, FAAN, is the nurse scientist manager for the department of nursing at Arkansas Children's Hospital, Little Rock, Arkansas. She is also adjunct associate professor in the College of Nursing at the University of Arkansas for Medical Sciences, Little Rock, Arkansas. Dr. Walden's program of research is pain in preterm neonates, and she has successfully competed for both foundation and federal grants to advance her program of research. Dr. Walden received an R21 grant to explore the effects of light, sound, and sleep on pain responses in preterm neonates. She has taught research and grant writing at the graduate level, but her passion is teaching and mentoring clinical nurses in evidence-based practice and research.

• • •

Grant Writing Handbook for Nurses and Health Professionals

Third Edition

Barbara J. Holtzclaw, PhD, RN, FAAN
Carole Kenner, PhD, RN, FAAN, FNAP, ANEF
Marlene Walden, PhD, APRN, NNP-BC, CCNS, FAAN

SPRINGER PUBLISHING COMPANY

Springer Publishing Company, LLC
11 West 42nd Street
New York, NY 10036
www.springerpub.com

Acquisitions Editor: Margaret Zuccarini
Associate Managing Editor: Kris Parrish
Compositor: S4Carlisle

ISBN: 978-0-8261-4144-6
ebook ISBN: 978-0-8261-4145-3
Instructor's PowerPoints ISBN: 978-0-8261-4146-0

Instructor's Materials: Qualified instructors may request supplements by emailing textbook@ springerpub.com

18 19 20 21 22 / 5 4 3 2 1

The author and the publisher of this Work have made every effort to use sources believed to be reliable to provide information that is accurate and compatible with the standards generally accepted at the time of publication. The author and publisher shall not be liable for any special, consequential, or exemplary damages resulting, in whole or in part, from the readers' use of, or reliance on, the information contained in this book. The publisher has no responsibility for the persistence or accuracy of URLs for external or third-party Internet websites referred to in this publication and does not guarantee that any content on such websites is, or will remain, accurate or appropriate.

Library of Congress Cataloging-in-Publication Data

Names: Holtzclaw, Barbara J., author. | Kenner, Carole, author. | Walden,
   Marlene, 1956- author.
Title: Grant writing handbook for nurses and health professionals / Barbara
   J. Holtzclaw, Carole Kenner, Marlene Walden.
Other titles: Grant writing handbook for nurses
Description: Third edition. | New York : Springer Publishing Company, [2018]
   | Preceded by Grant writing handbook for nurses / Barbara J. Holtzclaw,
   Carole Kenner, Marlene Walden. 2nd ed. c2001. | Includes bibliographical
   references and index.
Identifiers: LCCN 2017058491| ISBN 9780826141446 | ISBN 9780826141453 (ebook)
   | ISBN 9780826141460 (instructor's PowerPoints)
Subjects: | MESH: Research Support as Topic | Nursing Research | Writing |
   Fellowships and Scholarships--standards
Classification: LCC RT81.5 | NLM WY 20.5 | DDC 610.73072--dc23 LC record available at
https://lccn.loc.gov/2017058491

Printed in the United States of America.

Contents

Preface

Relatively few nurses or healthcare professionals enter their area of practice with an idea of writing a grant. Even those seeking advanced clinical training or degrees may overlook the possibility. Yet many of the goals and realities of a meaningful career require nurses and clinicians in all disciplines to request funding for projects that focus on education, clinical practice, research, or a combination of these. Grant writing is an essential skill for nursing and health scientists today but one we receive little training for, even in advanced graduate programs. So, where do you start? Where do you look for guidance? Where do you find foundations or agencies that fund enterprises like yours? These questions tend to be of first concern to most new grant writers. However, as you sit at the keyboard to write the grant, you may also feel somewhat intimidated by unfamiliar terminology, puzzling forms, and the variety of submission formats required by funding agencies. This process is more frustrating if you are unfamiliar with the structure, conventions, and essential elements of grant preparation. This grant writing handbook is a very informal conversation about the art of proposing and the process of writing grants with minimal frustration. At least we hope we accomplish that goal!

Each of the authors is an experienced grant writer, grant reviewer, and grantsmanship consultant. Examples include tips from their grant writing workshops and experiences from their own projects. The book is formatted to follow the basic steps of grant writing. We have written it in the first person to get the reader involved in the process. You will find other books on writing fundable grants that are very detailed, grant-specific, and devoid of real-life experiences. We attempted to cut to the chase and give you bare-bones strategies and quick tips that a busy professional—a would-be grant writer—needs for this adventure. In this edition, updates on electronic submissions, new grant funding areas, and web resources have been added. A new chapter (Chapter 6) highlights changes in how researchers need to engage with community stakeholders from grant development through implementation. **Qualified instructors may obtain access to ancillary instructor's PowerPoints by emailing textbook@springerpub.com.**

Grant writing can be exciting and even profitable given the right tools. This book is one of the "right tools." Happy grant writing!

Barbara J. Holtzclaw
Carole Kenner
Marlene Walden

Acknowledgments

We would like to thank Margaret Zuccarini and Elizabeth Nieginski at Springer Publishing Company for supporting the third edition. The original project grew out of a presentation done by Drs. Carole Kenner and Marlene Walden at a National Association of Neonatal Nurses (NANN) conference. This edition includes content from grantsmanship workshops presented by Dr. Barbara Holtzclaw at national and regional conferences and for nursing and interdisciplinary faculty-development programs in Texas, Oklahoma, Alabama, and North Carolina.

We gratefully acknowledge the consultation and insight regarding community-engaged health research in Chapter 6, "Engaging Communities in Research Grant Development," provided by Pamela Holtzclaw Williams, JD, PhD, RN, during her appointment as associate professor, College of Nursing, University of Arkansas for Medical Sciences, Graduate Program. Dr. Williams served as principal investigator on three community engagement–funded studies and projects funded by the Patient-Centered Outcome Research Institute (PCORI) and served as a PCORI study section member. She was actively involved with community-engagement initiatives and funding by Clinical and Translational Science Awards at several academic health science centers. She serves as an ambassador for PCORI and consults on funded engagement projects.

1

. . .

Why Grant Writing Skills Are Needed Now and in the Future

. . .

WHAT IS YOUR GRANT WRITING INCENTIVE?

Perhaps your incentive to write a grant may have come from a deep-seated desire to be a grant writer. If so, you are unusual and have an interesting life's work cut out for you. However, for the rest of us, and the majority of health professionals, the motivation to write a grant comes from a need to finance a project, a study, or an educational program. In fact, many persons in healthcare find writing a grant a completely new experience. Even those who have received advanced degrees may not have training or experience in seeking funds for their projects. Also, if unfamiliarity with grantsmanship makes grant writing seem overwhelming and intimidating, remember that it is a *learned skill* and one that draws on your existing abilities and talents. If that is where you are beginning, it is worthwhile to resist the "means to an end" view of looking for expediency rather than a good fit with an idea and a potential funding agency. Taking the long view of grant-proposal writing involves realizing that these skills can be used again and again. Acquaintance with today's rapidly changing professional demands and economic conditions emphasizes the urgency for prospective strategies and skills for successful grant writing. Changing priorities and funding initiatives also emphasize the importance of keeping updated on these changes and knowing where to look for them. This chapter addresses a few of the important demands and constraints that make strategic grantsmanship essential.

Increasingly, many faculty, administrators, or project coordinators in healthcare settings find that job security depends on the art of grant writing. Therefore, grant writing is not a skill for the select few who seek this as their life's work; it is an essential form of communication for healthcare professionals across a diverse spectrum of positions. It is to be taken seriously as something you can add to your already-developed set of communication skills. Acquiring solid grant writing knowledge means learning some new language, conventions, processes, and skills that will enable you to be successful in an increasingly competitive funding market. Because change is always expected, your ongoing success will depend on maintaining a steady stream of current information from funding sources.

• • •

NATIONAL TRENDS DRIVE THE NEED AND BOOST THE COMPETITION FOR FUNDING

Competition for grant funds has increased appreciably in response to several national trends that go beyond the expected rise and fall of economic conditions. Here are a few trends that directly drive the need for grant funding but, at the same time, tend to make competition for funds stiffer.

NIH Roadmap

A major funding initiative introduced in 2002 continues to influence funding as institutes began to collaborate more closely. The roadmap was conceived when the director of the National Institutes of Health (NIH) convened leaders in academia, industry, government, and the public, to chart a plan for medical research in the 21st century. The initiative came from a growing recognition that individual disciplines and single NIH institutes could not tackle major opportunities and gaps in biomedical research alone. In 2004, plans for the NIH Roadmap for Medical Research emerged to engage all of the NIH entities in the process of transforming and translating new and developing scientific knowledge more quickly into "tangible benefits" for the health of people. With the 2006 NIH Reform Act, Congress enacted the NIH Common Fund into law to support cross-cutting, trans-NIH programs. Grant applications require participation, strategic planning, and coordination with at least two NIH entities (NIH, 2015). This meant not only moving research findings from bench to bedside more quickly, but also forming new relationships across disciplines, including nursing. The three areas of emphasis included new pathways to discovery, research teams of the future, and re-engineering the clinical research enterprise. "Translational research" became the goal of training efforts, collaborative studies, and coordination activities. Although the goals and outcomes of the NIH Roadmap were easily embraced, its implementation offered new challenges and a need for scientists to interact differently. The NIH recognized the need for broad reengineering to bring about a new discipline of clinical and translational science. The Clinical and Translational Science Awards (CTSA) Consortium was launched in 2006, and initially 12 academic health centers were funded with competitive CTSA awards. Now there are over 60 centers. Other institutions competed for planning grants. The influence of the NIH Roadmap and translational research remains evident in the National Institute of Nursing Research (NINR) agenda and translational science initiatives and promotion of collaborations across institutes. These emphases are seen in published current NIH funding opportunities for developing Big Data to Knowledge, Discovery of Genetic Basis of Childhood Cancers and Structural Birth Defects, and Health Care Systems Research (NIH, 2016). Priorities for translational research are reflected in NIH application instructions for research and training grants. Whereas this trend offers new hope for faster translation of science into action and greater interdisciplinary, transdisciplinary, and cross-disciplinary research, it also introduces a variety of new complexities in shared support, budgetary, subcontract, and oversight that are discussed in later chapters.

NIH Common Fund and the American Recovery and Reinvestment Act

In 2010, the development of novel NIH Common Fund awards enabled by the new American Recovery and Reinvestment Act (ARRA) brought about funding of unique and highly innovative studies believed to have potential to "accelerate discovery in biomedicine and development of new treatments for myriad diseases and disorders." Whereas these grants are currently funding a variety of "omics"-focused projects (e.g., metabolomics, epigenetics, genomic influences on childhood cancer, interactions between drugs and the genome), new initiatives are expected to emerge to fund large-scale, novel, and cutting-edge studies to achieve more rapid discovery (NIH, 2016).

Patient-Centered Outcomes Research Institute

The independent nonprofit, nongovernmental organization, Patient-Centered Outcomes Research Institute (PCORI), was authorized by Congress in 2010 through the Patient Protection and Affordable Care Act and funded through the Patient-Centered Outcomes Research Trust Fund (PCOR Trust Fund). PCORI is designed to help patients, families, and clinicians address health problems with reliable information and clinical effectiveness in ways that help them make care decisions. They funded comparative clinical effectiveness research to provide evidence for care decisions. PCORI was established with a clear mandate to carry out the funding of comparative clinical effectiveness research (PCORI, 2016). Community engagement of care recipients and care providers has been an essential element for this funding in which patients and other stakeholders are the primary stimulus for initiatives. Often, but not always, engagement of these stakeholders is required when a proposal is submitted. Funding initiatives are based on emerging high-priority topics and research questions identified by patients, informal caregivers, clinicians, or healthcare delivery systems. A highly informative training system for PCORI grant applicants includes online training, online instruction for submission of letter of intent and application, and webinar "town hall" meetings to discuss cycle-specific points. Because there is a learning-curve to building capacity and engaging community around a common research goal, "pipeline awards" are available to support beginning partnerships. Tier I pipeline awards fund seed grants, whereas Tiers II and III offer increasingly higher amounts to allow the research team to build toward full PCORI funding announcements in which the major emphasis is on studies that compare clinical effectiveness, risks, and benefits of two or more healthcare approaches, and studies that improve methods available for clinical effectiveness research. Of high priority are studies that involve conditions affecting large numbers of diverse populations and those that place heavy care burdens on individuals, families, and specific populations; the community; and society. Populations of interest include racial/ethnic minorities; women; children; older adults; those from rural areas; low-income people; people with limited health literacy; lesbian, gay, bisexual, and transgender (LGBT) persons; veterans and armed forces members and families; and individuals with special healthcare needs, disabilities, multiple chronic diseases, rare diseases, and genetically acquired medical conditions (PCORI, 2016). The close association between PCORI and the Patient Protection and Affordable Care Act raised some uncertainty regarding its continued funding following the 2016 national elections that influenced congressional support. However, PCORI funding from the PCOR Trust Fund receives income from three funding streams: the general fund appropriations of the U.S. Treasury, transfers from the Centers for Medicare & Medicaid trust funds, and a fee assessed on private insurance and the PCOR fee paid by self-insured health plans (PCORI, 2016).

The enthusiasm for the goals and the perceived impact of patient-centered outcomes and comparative clinical effectiveness outcomes will continue to influence other funding agencies. The clinical effectiveness of patient-centered outcomes can be seen in federal funding opportunities from the NIH, the Agency for Healthcare Research and Quality (AHRQ), and others (U.S. National Library of Medicine, 2017).

The Magnet® Hospital Movement

As the name suggests, a "Magnet" hospital is one that can attract and retain nurses. During the staffing crisis of the early 1980s, the American Academy of Nursing found that hospitals with the best record of staffing met a common set of criteria that exemplified quality care. The *Magnet Hospital* movement was developed a decade later in 1994 by the American Nurses Credentialing Center (ANCC). This initiative recognizes healthcare organizations that provide nursing excellence. To compete for excellent staff and recognition of excellence, nurse administrators engage in research efforts to identify nursing care problems and measure nurse-sensitive indicators of quality in their agency. Nurse administrators, in turn, also encourage bedside nurses to perform unit-based research and evidence-based practice (EBP) projects and to apply for seed grants from foundations or practice organizations. The process of validating the effectiveness of nursing and medical therapies has become a concern of clinical staff, as well as the academicians in health science centers and nursing organizations.

Quests for Funding to Demonstrate Nurse-Sensitive Quality Care

In 1994, the American Nurses Association (ANA) launched a safety and quality initiative, seeking links between nursing care and patient outcomes that led to several competitive grant writing invitations for proposals. Projects funded from this initiative began with "Nursing Care Report Card for Acute Care," "National Database of Nursing Quality Indicators," and finally an award in 2001 to the Midwest Research Institute (MRI) and the University of Kansas School of Nursing to manage the ANA'S National Database of Nursing Quality Indicators (NDNQI). NDNQI funded early pilot studies from 1997 to 2000 to test nurse-sensitive quality indicators and established a system for collecting and providing comparative information to healthcare facilities for use in quality improvement activities. In 2001, they developed a fee-based process of data submission and comparison reports. Today, more than 2,000 U.S. hospitals and 98% of Magnet recognized facilities or hospitals participate in NDNQI'S program and contribute data to a growing national database that is available to qualified researchers for studying the relationship between nurse staffing and patient outcomes (NDNQI, 2016). This trend has not only engaged hospitals in the process of seeking best practices, but also generated a movement toward testing new interventions to improve nurse-sensitive quality outcomes. Likewise, the national quest for improved quality by the CMS and the ARRA has provided funding incentives and recognition for healthcare providers and hospitals to adopt certified electronic health records to facilitate data collection and monitoring of health quality measures (Dykes & Collins, 2013).

EBP Movement

The EBP movement has raised interest and funding activity around the develop-ment and testing of research-based protocols. EBP has stimulated organizations and hospitals to offer seed grants for unit-based studies that test best practice nursing intervention protocols. The movement to base clinical nursing practice on research findings causes many to confuse EBP with "research utilization" (RU). Although both embrace some of the same philosophic underpinnings, EBP goes beyond the review, critique, and application of scientific research that characterizes RU. Sackett, Rosenberg, Gray, Haynes, & Richardson (1996) define EBP as "the conscientious, explicit and judicious use of current best evidence in making decisions about the care of individual patients." The quality-filtering aspect of seeking best evidence requires expertise on the part of clinicians and researchers to find and review relevant literature, weigh its merit to provide "best evidence," and finally to consider the patient's preferences and values to guide care. The EBP movement has engaged nearly every health profession, and each group struggles with issues of integrating newly emerging discoveries into practice decisions. Preparing nurses to participate fully in the quality-filtering enterprise requires many to receive additional training. Still other nurses rely on evidence-based medicine databases, such as the Cochrane Reviews, or infor-mation sheets for best nursing practice, such as those provided by the Joanna Briggs Institute. These well-developed databases provide evidence reports that are based on rigorous, comprehensive syntheses and analyses of the scientific literature. There is a level of excitement about EBP among nurses who found their research course in nursing school difficult or boring. Some view EBP as a way to improve clinical practice without engaging in the rigor or preparation of conducting research. However, all should realize that nursing research is still the foundation for providing the scientific basis for the "evidence" in EBP. Finding nursing research on a specific problem or intervention and weighing its merit is only possible if such research evidence exists. Mitchell (2006) points out this as a disparity and challenges the profession to improve the culture that nurtures well-prepared, research-active practitioners. Although well-planned research investigations are increasing the knowledge base, there remains a significant gap in providing sufficient evidence to meet our present and future needs.

The Move to Electronic Extramural Grant Submission

The electronic age has made an unusual impact on the grant writing enterprise, and with rare exceptions, all federal extramural grants must be received as elec-tronic documents incorporated in established electronic forms. The movement to web-based electronic grant proposal submission has required a remarkable increase in computer skills for grant writers and secretarial support. At the same time, it has required a competent infrastructure in support services and personnel from universities, hospitals, and organizations. Although these changes are most evident in the application process of the NIH and other federal funding agencies, small practice and professional organizations are also moving to electronic submissions. Electronic submission processes are discussed more fully in later chapters.

Quests for Extramural Funding for Conference Support

As nursing has grown in absolute numbers and consciousness of its role and power to exert widespread change, so has the need for support for large conferences, summits, and think tanks. The costs for large meetings of this sort can be beyond a single institution or group's capability, so many turn to extramural funding to pay for meeting sites, speakers, and in some cases, travel for attendees. Foundations, such as the American Nurses Foundation (ANF), or agencies, such as the AHRQ, have funded grants for such meetings. Other agencies fund conferences that disseminate important information. For example, Substance Abuse and Mental Health Services Administration (SAMHSA) Center for Mental Health Services (CMHS), Center for Substance Abuse Prevention (CSAP), and Center for Substance Abuse Treatment (CSAT) fund grants to disseminate knowledge about practices in mental health services and substance abuse prevention and treatment. Awareness of the possibilities for conference funding may exist within your own organizations, so a well-crafted grant proposal for this purpose may be in your future.

*   *   *

RISING LEVEL OF PREPARATION FOR CLINICAL NURSE LEADERS COMPETING FOR GRANTS

Advanced practice nurses and nurse administrators in clinical settings quickly realize that grant writing is not just an activity for their colleagues in the ivory tower of nursing research and education. They find that grant writing skills are a necessity as healthcare moves toward implementing EBP and nurse-sensitive quality evaluation. Managed care contracts emphasize evidence of cost-effective, outcome-based care through standardization of clinical protocols and treatment plans. Care maps have become benchmark processes in the care of specific patient populations. As hospital-based nurses face these rigorous challenges for validating standards of care, they lack the personnel or financial resources to do so. Clinical nurse leaders are realizing the necessity for advanced preparation in writing proposals and designing projects with measurable outcomes. Several nursing organizations have responded to their members' need for skills in grantsmanship and offer workshops on proposal writing. Doctoral programs that prepare nursing administrators have begun to include grant writing as part of career training. Hospitals have engaged faculty from academic institutions to provide consultation to their nurse leaders as they write grants to support important clinical practice priorities. A growing trend is for hospitals and clinical agencies to employ nurse scientists with research training who can provide assistance in setting up well-designed projects and evaluation plans.

● ● ●

NURSING SHORTAGE HEIGHTENS THE NEED FOR EDUCATORS AS FUNDS DWINDLE

Several economic trends have affected the need to seek external funding for educational training programs and research. As money becomes scarcer for agencies and institutions, positions and programs are threatened. Training and demonstration grants have traditionally been resources that keep important programs afloat until better times. However, widespread economic deficits have spread these grant funds thin. At the same time, nationwide cuts in general employment tend to increase the numbers of applicants to healthcare programs because laid-off workers return to school seeking second careers. The trickle-down effects of raising funds to sustain educational programs while applicant pools swell is magnified only by the need for faculty to teach in these programs. Faculty, in turn, must maintain a program of research and scholarship to be seriously considered for promotion and tenure. Institutions that once may have granted these attributes to good teachers without programs of research have raised the bar. Grant writing is an expectation for funding the research or demonstration project that will yield publications and demonstrate scholarly merit. Funding agencies and granting foundations have dealt with the tremendous increase in grant applications in a fair, but highly competitive, manner. They too have raised the bar by requiring applicants to meet stiffer criteria and engaging experts in the field to review grant proposals.

● ● ●

RISING RAPID PROLIFERATION OF DOCTORAL PROGRAMS REQUIRE PROGRAM AND TRAINING SUPPORT

The need for more nursing faculty at all levels has stimulated the proliferation of doctoral programs. Yet it is surprising how little instruction is spent on grantsmanship in an educational program to prepare nursing faculty. Even with the advance of nursing science, research-focused doctoral programs, and the growing numbers of nurses involved in research, they tend to receive little formal training on seeking funding for their work. In university settings, faculty members soon become aware that successful grantsmanship is a valued step toward promotion, tenure status, and/or continued employment at a particular academic or clinical institution. Faculty are under great pressure to write research grants to develop, revise, or expand their own programs of research and to write program-training grants to meet changing student, institutional, or managed care demands that affect educational programs.

* * *

CONSTRAINTS IN FEDERAL FUNDING FOR RESEARCH WHILE DEMANDS FOR FUNDS INCREASE

No research-funding agency has felt the economic pinch more than the U.S. federal government. Funds, allocated by the U.S. Congress, are lobbied for competitively by each of its institutes, centers, and divisions. The U.S. Public Health Service houses several of the major competitors for federal funds. These include the Administration for Children and Families (ACF), Administration for Community Living (ACL), AHRQ, Agency for Toxic Substances and Disease Registry (ATSDR), Centers for Disease Control and Prevention (CDC), CMS, Food and Drug Administration (FDA), Health Resources & Services Administration (HRSA), Indian Health Service (IHS), NIH, and SAMHSA. Even the relatively new Nursing Common Fund and the ARRA-funded PCORI entities vary in appropriations with changes in national, social, and political priorities. The NIH, a major funding agency for nursing research, has seen a decline in federal research spending as national priorities of defense and biodefense take precedent. Despite the rising need for research funds, the future for funding is uncertain. A bipartisan agreement boosted funding in 2017 despite proposed cuts to the biomedical science budget. However, as appropriation proposals for 2018 became clear, severe slashing of the entire NIH budget, along with possible cuts to programs, offices, and agencies, was predicted (Kaiser, 2017; Rosseter, 2017). According to the American Association of Colleges of Nursing, such deep cuts to the national centers for healthcare research are unprecedented (Rosseter, 2017). Nursing research remains a low funding priority despite evidence of outstanding contributions, particularly in the area of women's health and geriatric research. Although the need for activism to support federal research funding may seem distant from your early efforts in grant writing, all citizens have a voice in encouraging support of federal funding for healthcare research. Your voice is important as both a healthcare professional and a research scientist at any level. The Friends of the National Institute for Nursing Research (FNINR) is an active effort on the part of nursing to raise funds to lobby Congress to increase funding in this area.

● ● ●

NEED FOR INCREASED COMPETENCIES AND NEW GRANT WRITING INFRASTRUCTURE

The days of liberal funding are over, and as waning funds boost competition for grant funds it raises the bar for acceptable quality of grant proposals. No longer can nursing deans and administrators casually expect of their employees, "While you're up, get me a grant!" Instead, thoughtful nurse leaders are recognizing the need to provide support and training to new faculty and key clinical leaders. Some nursing schools are implementing "nurse scholars" programs with light teaching loads for selected faculty who are being trained in grantsmanship by the institution's research dean and designates. Others encourage faculty to seek postdoctoral training and career awards to improve competencies in research and grantsmanship. Finally, the complexity of maintaining a "well-oiled machine" for providing support and consultation to faculty or nursing staff who submit grants has led many institutions to create a grant writing infrastructure with writing, statistical, and budgetary consultation, including oversight of the compilation and submission of federal forms.

CONCLUSION

Grant writing is an expectation of many nurses, healthcare providers, and affiliated support professionals, whether they are in academia or clinical settings. Increasingly, staders and volunteers in community engagement are being expected to contribute to the grant writing mission. Although funding for research or educational projects is tight, taking time to think through your project and then seeking a funding source whose mission is aligned with the project increase the chances of a successful grant application.

REFERENCES

Dykes, P., & Collins, S. (2013). Building linkages between nursing care and improved patient outcomes: The role of health information technology. *OJIN: The Online Journal of Issues in Nursing, 18*(3), 4. doi:10.1186/1748-5908-5-32

Kaiser, J. (2017). NIH overhead plan draws fire. *Science, 356*(6341), 893. doi:10.1112/science.356.6341.893

Mitchell, P. H. (2006). Research and development in nursing revisited: Nursing science as the basis for evidence-based practice. *Journal of Advanced Nursing, 54*(5), 528–529. doi:10.1111/j.1365-2648.2006.03852_3.x

National Database of Nursing Quality Indicators. (2016). Nursing quality (NDNQI): Improve care quality, prevent adverse events with deep nursing quality insights. Retrieved from http://www.pressganey.com/solutions/clinical-quality/nursing-quality

National Institutes of Health. (2015). About the NIH Common Fund. Retrieved from https://commonfund.nih.gov/about

National Institutes of Health. (2016). New program features. Retrieved from https://commonfund.nih.gov

Patient-Centered Outcomes Research Institute. (2016). Our programs. Retrieved from http://www.pcori.org/about-us/our-programs

Rosseter, R. (2017). Debilitating cuts proposed to research, workforce, and health programs [Press release]. Retrieved from http://www.businesswire.com/news/home/20170316005953/en/AACN-Strongly-Opposes-Presidents-2018-Budget-Blueprint

Sackett, D. L., Rosenberg, W. M., Gray, J. A., Haynes, R. B., & Richardson, W. S. (1996). Evidence-based medicine: What it is and what it isn't. *British Journal of Medicine, 312*, 71–72. doi:10.1136/bmj.312.7023.71

U.S. National Library of Medicine. (2017). Health Services Research Information Central: Comparative Effectiveness Research (CER). Retrieved from https://www.nlm.nih.gov/hsrinfo/cer.html#1026News:%20Comparative%20Effectiveness%20Research

2

So, You Want to Write a Grant! Where to Begin?

DEVELOPING A COMPELLING PROPOSAL!

Like any worthwhile endeavor, the process of grant writing is time-consuming. At times it may feel all-encompassing, with a life of its own. However, getting a grant funded is also doable, given the right idea and some basic grant writing skills. Breaking down the project into manageable pieces is often the key to success. This chapter focuses on developing the approach to or "art" of proposing, finding sources by which to generate fundable ideas, and finally, how to know if you are asking the right question. Although many types of grants are available, three of the most common include *research*, *program/training*, and *special projects/demonstration*. Examples in this chapter primarily address the research grant, although the majority of grant writing principles may apply to other types of grants.

THE FINE ART OF PROPOSING

There is an art to requesting someone to give something of value to you. There should be something inherently desirable that you can offer to the party from whom you are requesting funds. A proposal is a formal kind of request, whether it is for someone's hand in marriage or for funds for a research or training grant. If the marriage comparison seems a little absurd, remember that both situations involve requests to convince a person or persons to form a relationship and both require commitments and outcomes in return for the exchange. Acknowledging these similarities can help you recognize the need to make abundantly clear the following points in your proposal:

- Is the relationship relevant?
- Is the partner capable?
- Is the partner reliable?
- Can the partner be trusted with money?
- Does the partner present a neat, attractive, positive, and innovative image?
- Does the partner pay attention to schedules and time agreements?

Specifically, each element of a successful proposal must convincingly present and justify your desirability as a partner to your funding agency. Grant reviewers look at different aspects of your proposal to determine how well your plan, your training and experience, and your overall presentation reflect these points. A successful research proposal accomplishes the following four objectives:

1. Ask a meaningful question that is relevant to the funding agency.
2. Use good science that is novel and innovative to answer the question.
3. Pay careful attention to the application.
4. Demonstrate that the applicant is qualified to carry out the proposed project.

Table 2.1 explains how the elements of a successful proposal relate to the types of information that must be included.

● ● ●

THE MEANINGFUL QUESTION

A meaningful question has relevance to something of importance to the funding agency. Few funding sources are anxious to provide support to fill a gap in knowledge just because it is empty. In fact, many organizations or agencies offering grants have specific initiatives or priorities that must be addressed in your proposal's purpose and aims. Therefore, you should *clearly conceptualize* the question or knowledge gap you are proposing to address by your project. Articulate the outcomes of your project in the form of *clearly stated aims*. Write your study aims in specific, measurable terms (that is why they are called *specific aims*) and avoid using the "shotgun" approach of using generalities.

Grant reviewers look for a "flow" in proposals. This flow is not just a grammatical flow, but also one between your work as a scientist and the way that the proposed study fits with your future plans. Reviewers find helpful a statement clarifying links between your proposed project and your past and future program of research and scholarship. Likewise, a logical flow between your proposed

TABLE 2.1

ELEMENTS OF A SUCCESSFUL PROPOSAL

The Meaningful Question	
Articulates the following:	**Is supported by these characteristics**
• What will we learn from your research? • Why is it important to have the answer? • Is there a reasonable expectation that we will get the answer? • Why is the answer important to the funding agency?	• Clear sense of long-term scientific objectives • Rationale for need clearly linked to current state of the science • Evidence of thorough understanding of current research and literature • Relevance to the funding agency's priorities and congruence with its philosophies

Good Science	
Articulates the following:	**Supported by these characteristics**
• Thorough planning	• Conceptual and methodological links between each section are clear.
• Rationale for selected methods	• Every approach, method, instrument, and analytic step is clearly justified.
• Adequate description of methods	• Complex or new procedures, protocols, devices, and instruments are clarified with description, citations, and schematics.
• Clearly stated assumptions and limitations	• Assumptions, potential biases, and study limitations are clearly articulated.
• Identified problems and anticipated solutions	• Potential problems and factors affecting recruitment, retention, and protocol are acknowledged with possible solutions, including novel approaches to overcome past research challenges or new data-collection methods.
• Power calculations	• Sample size is based on statistically sound power calculations that take into consideration the postulated effect size that emerged from previous studies. Free power calculators are available online; however, your statistical consultant should help you understand the need to do more than crunch numbers.

(continued)

TABLE 2.1

ELEMENTS OF A SUCCESSFUL PROPOSAL (*continued*)

Careful Attention to the Application

Articulates the following:	Supported by these characteristics
• Compliance with instructions	• Proposal is submitted with proper format, with supporting documents, and on time.
• Clear, lucid writing style	• Proposal is written in a clear, active voice and jargon-free style, with no run-on sentences.
• Neat appearance	• Text, graphics, and tables are orderly and consistently organized.
• Grammatically and typographically correct	• Careful proofreading, grammar-check, and spell-checking of proposal and references are performed.
• Proper type size	• Careful attention is paid to font type and size.
• Appropriate use of appendices	• There is compliance with the number and the indexing of appendices in the proposal.

Qualified Applicant

Articulates the following:	Supported by these characteristics
• Showing your familiarity with the topic	• Prior research and publications reflect interest in and familiarity with the topic.
• Showing understanding of the methods	• Methods are justified in detail to explain testing for outcomes.
• Demonstrating ability to carry out the planned study	• Biosketch, pilot, and preliminary work reflect knowledge of research skill, previous funding, and research partners.

Source: Primary elements adapted from a presentation by Dr. June Lunney, NINR/NIH, at Southern Nursing Research Society Annual Conference, 11th Annual Research Conference, February 1997, Norfolk, VA.

project and the funding organization's priorities helps establish the relevance of the project. Tables or outlines can also demonstrate links between the project's broad goals, the narrower purpose or purposes, and the specific aims and related questions or hypotheses. As you develop the proposal, your description of the sampling frame, methods chosen, and plan for analysis or evaluation must follow a logical progression to measure how well the aims are achieved. For quantitative research proposals, the proposal usually includes plans to demonstrate achievement of specific aims through tests of hypotheses, analyses of costs and benefits, and clear descriptions of previously unknown phenomena. Qualitative research studies also have expected outcomes, but the nature of the inquiry, methodology, and data collection produces outcomes that are inductively analyzed for meaning, categorizations, and description. A qualitative research proposal can stay true to its inductive roots, but have a higher likelihood of meeting funding priorities if you can (a) justify how the information you will gain can achieve the specific aims and (b) state how it will help meet the broad goals of the study.

EMPLOYING GOOD SCIENCE

We have established that writing a scientifically sound proposal requires sufficient knowledge about a topic to ask meaningful questions. It is just as important to write a convincing proposal showing that you are likely to get meaningful answers to these questions during your study. This process involves the science of research. First of all, your research design deserves thought and consultation from an expert. Getting outside help to confirm or suggest alternatives to your design is time and possible expense that may save you considerable rearranging and distress later. The design should be selected and justified to show a reviewer that the approach you have selected is the best possible approach for answering the specific question and achieving the specific aim. Finding support for a particular approach in the literature is often excellent rationale to be included (and cited) in the proposal. You will need to follow the process of justifying each different question and aim, which may or may not have a similar rationale or approach.

This is the place where innovations in research methods, theoretical concepts, or interventions need to be addressed. Innovation implies not only newness, but also a sense of unique utility. Innovation is proposing to solve a problem in new ways by either generating new ideas or applying existing ideas to a new situation that results in the improvement of healthcare outcomes.

Many grants, including research grants, seek novel or innovative ways to tackle a problem. The National Institutes of Health (NIH) Application Guide to Grants and Funding Information includes a section where the applicant must identify the significance and innovation. See the NIH website for more information (NIH, 2018).

One example of innovation is seen in an NIH working group report on an innovative way to address obesity and the maintenance of weight loss (MacLean et al., 2015). They conclude that research physiologists and other researchers need to look at the multitiered problem of excess weight and the maintenance of weight loss and that new combinations of drugs and therapies must be examined (MacLean et al., 2015). Tailoring approaches at the individual level is another novel approach and supports the move toward personalized health.

Innovation often involves putting together existing interventions in a novel or new way. Innovation may include new methodologies or a new look at an old topic. For example, in the 1990s, transition to care was a hot topic. It is again today, but the novel approach addresses care coordination, costs associated with transitional care models, reimbursement for services, and impact on rehospitalizations. The work is population based, looking at the elderly, premature infants, and preoperative, intraoperative, and postoperative care, for example. The framework has stayed over the years, but the aspects of transitions have broadened to reflect changes in healthcare practices domestically and globally. Instruments for measurement, for example, have evolved into a tool for parents of premature infants and their transition from hospital to home (Boykova, 2016).

Research is also shifting to more outcomes that often include quality care and patient safety. This change represents a paradigm shift in the foci of research, especially clinically based research. Research has also shifted to include more web-based survey techniques, leading to global studies, as well as use of the large data sets now available at the state, national, and global levels. For example, New Jersey has the Big Data Alliance data set that can be used as deidentified data to examine health trends (see njbda.weebly.com).

• • •

JUSTIFYING MEASUREMENT INSTRUMENTS AND DEVICES

Describing the choice of instruments or measurement devices may also require some help from experts or colleagues who have access to or familiarity with your selected method. For instruments with psychometric properties, getting reliability and validity estimates on similar types of research participants may be possible from the literature or directly from the author or developer. If you plan to use the instrument to measure variables in a study with a different type, age, or situational group, testing it on a sample from your proposed group will strengthen your proposal. Particular attention should be given to estimating the feasibility, validity, and reliability of instruments when using them with persons who do not speak English as their first language and in persons with temporary or progressive cognitive impairment. Many psychosocial instruments were normed from tests done with college-age students, so you should seek documentation or demonstrate that the instrument is relevant to the age or developmental capabilities of your study subjects.

• • •

JUSTIFYING BIOLOGICAL MEASURES

Measurement devices, medical instruments, biological assays, and tissue samples are being incorporated more often in nursing care studies. Although they may be mystifying and appear to have a scientific objectivity to the lay public, funding agencies usually engage reviewers with the background to know or easily find the sensitivity, precision, accuracy, reliability, and appropriateness of such measures. Therefore, it is a measure of "good science" to articulate and justify the ability and the limits of the biological test you intend to use. In some cases, you may need to justify the use of a new assay that replaces a previously unreliable one. Consider including a brief "mini-tutorial" in your justification to help you pose and resolve an objection before the reviewer does. Along with justification, it is wise for new investigators to show availability and involvement of consultants and experts as they use new or complex instrumentation. Omitting your access to expertise does not make you appear wiser. On the contrary, even experts seek higher certainty and assurance.

● ● ●

JUSTIFYING STEPS FOR DATA COLLECTION

Procedures and protocols can get complicated, particularly if you are using one design to test one specific aim and a different design to test another aim. Using a diagram is helpful for showing the variations in a complex protocol. Figure 2.1 is an example of a diagram depicting a comparison of

FIGURE 2.1 Using a diagram to explain a complex design.

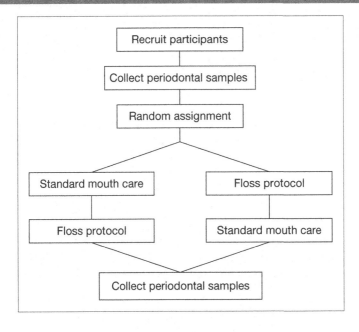

persons infected with HIV to determine if an established flossing protocol done before or after mouth care was associated with less residual debris in periodontal pockets.

. . .

JUSTIFYING STATISTICAL APPROACHES

Determining the appropriate statistics to use is always a concern in proposal development. Here is another place where expert consultation is not only desirable, but also often essential. If you have clearly mapped your design, have identified your measurement variables, and know the nature of the data your instruments or measures will yield, the chore for you and your statistical consultant will be much easier. You will save considerable time with your consulting statistician if you get specific with *what, when,* and to *what degree of precision* you wish to measure each variable. Simply generalizing that you want to use blood pressure to measure stress or use hemoglobin A1c (HbA1c) to measure glucose control during pregnancy is a plan that is neither precise nor manageable enough to plan a statistical approach. Blood pressure measurements raise the questions, "Which ones (diastolic or systolic; standing or sitting; time of measurement)?" and "At what points during pregnancy will these variables be measured?" HbA1c use raises similar questions about which measurements will be used and whether you want to know exact levels, whether the levels will be meaningful without serial measures, or simply whether the patient was normoglycemic. If the latter is the case, you could possibly convert the numerical interval-level values of the variable HbA1c to ordinal-level variables such as hypoglycemic, normoglycemic, or hyperglycemic. The choice depends on the question, the design, and the availability of relational data. However, making a global statement such as "appropriate statistical tests" or "univariate and multivariate approaches" to explain data analyses leaves reviewers guessing if you actually understand what answers are possible from your planned analytic procedures.

. . .

JUSTIFYING SAMPLE SIZE

Seek consultation if you are unclear about how to justify your sample size. This is true of both qualitative and quantitative studies. Each approach has different guidelines underlying the choice. To show your familiarity with "good science," include the rationale for your choice.

Qualitative Sample Justification

There is an erroneous misconception among those less familiar with qualitative methods that sample size justification is not important. According to Sandelowski (1995), the sufficiency of a sample size for qualitative research has to do with its adequacy to perform the study's goal. In general, the quality, rather than the quantity, has been used in the past to justify and, sometimes, dodge the issue of sample size. Sandelowski's article points out that having too small or too large a sample can undermine a study. Knowledgeable grant reviewers understand this concept and expect you to justify a qualitative sample size. There is also a popular argument among scholars that the concept of saturation is the most important factor to consider (Dworkin, 2012). Even this guideline depends on how homogeneous or heterogeneous the population is and how important any demographic or conceptual differences are to the study. Although a relatively small sample of 10 might be adequate for homogeneous or critical case sampling, it would be too small to provide the variation needed to gather characteristics of a complex phenomenon. It would also be too small to develop theory. On the other hand, more is not always better, depending again on the study purpose. An extremely large sample is neither feasible nor desirable for conducting certain types of narrative analysis. Therefore, it is important to discuss and document the rationale for your choice.

Quantitative Sample Justification

The issues involved in justifying adequacy of sample size in quantitative research are aimed at (a) gaining a representative sample and (b) avoiding error. In general, a sample is more representative of a population if it contains more members. This makes sense because the smaller the sample, the greater the likelihood that you have missed members with various characteristics. The closer you get in size to the entire population, the less likely you are to miss members. However, it is usually not economically feasible or even necessary to include an entire population in a study. On the other hand, if the sample is too small, you may fail to detect a significant relationship (type II error). In justifying the sample size for a grant proposal, reviewers want to know the factors you have considered in arriving at that number. The gold standard for estimating the ability of a statistical test to detect a difference, if one exists, is a *power analysis*. Cohen (1988) developed the most frequently used method, which uses three parameters to calculate the power estimate. These include the *level of significance, desired power*, and *expected effect size*. The formula is not difficult, and the fact that power analyses can be readily done with certain computer programs has led many to simply choose arbitrary estimates of effect size, plug in the numbers, and "crunch" out a seemingly acceptable number for a power estimate. This is where a statistical consultant comes in handy to help you with the fine-tuning of the process. Although the first two parameters can be set by the investigator to avoid chances for error, the third parameter, the expected effect size, is determined by the "degree to which the phenomenon exists," as best you can determine (Cohen, 1988, p. 4). This is not just a wild guess or a desired level, but rather is an estimate based on preliminary data, pilot work, or existing studies found in the literature. According to Cohen, the degree of effect can be measured in a variety of ways that include "mean differences (raw or standardized), correlations and squared correlation of all kinds, odds ratios, kappas—whatever conveys the magnitude of the phenomenon of interest appropriate to the research context" (Cohen, 1990, p. 1310). Failing to estimate an accurate effect size might lead to incorrect conclusions about a study hypothesis because you might have a variable with such a small effect that a larger sample would be required to detect it. To make it clear to grant reviewers how you arrived at the effect size, indicate its source. Effect size is often misunderstood and one of the most often-ignored aspects of sample selection, yet its role in establishing your sample size is critical. Grant reviewers also want to know that you have considered *each proposed statistical test* you will use in the study in estimating the power. Different tables exist for estimating power, depending on the particular analysis, the numbers of groups, and the type of hypothesis (directional or nondirectional [which takes more subjects]). The sample size required to obtain the desired power will be different.

• • •

CAREFUL ATTENTION TO THE APPLICATION

The instructions for applying for a grant vary across funding agencies and organizations to the extent that nothing should be taken for granted. A useful exercise is to gather the application instructions from a printed or computer-generated source and begin marking it up with a colored highlighter marker. Highlight important facts that you will need to comply with to get your grant submitted in a timely, appropriately packaged form. For easy reference, it helps if you look for and highlight information related to the following:

- Requirements of a letter of intent and submission deadline. These are required for NIH grants and for many foundation grants for research and education. This letter of intent is a brief 2- to 10-page synopsis of the proposed area of study or educational program. The merits of such a letter determines whether a full proposal will be requested by the funding agency. NIH requests the title, contact information of the principal investigator,

key personnel, participating institutions, and the number and title of the funding call this letter involves (National Institute of Mental Health, 2016)
- Submission deadline, review, and award dates (include whether the submission date is the postmark date or the date of receipt by the agency)
- Name and address (or in some cases the e-mail address) to which the proposal is to be sent
- Page and space limitations for each section, as well as for the total grant proposal
- Type font size, margins, pagination, and reference style requirements
- Acceptability and limits on tables, figures, and appendices
- Budget page forms, budgetary limits, indirect cost limits, and modular requirements
- Acceptable categories or positions for key personnel, consultants, and services
- Limitations on salary for key personnel, consultants, and research assistants
- Limitations on travel, lodging, and support services
- Allowable expenses for equipment and supplies
- Requirements for biographical sketches, consultant information, and clinical agency clearances. For research training grants, clearances from supervisors or sponsors are required
- Requirements for institutional review board clearance before or after funding

This list varies depending on whether you are applying for a small seed grant or an extramural federal grant. However, the principles of carefully reviewing each and every requirement are essential in either case. Too often, grants are submitted in improper format, without proper documentation, or too late because the researcher failed to read the instructions closely. Nothing turns off a grant reviewer more than a sloppily organized grant proposal full of grammatical and spelling errors and with improperly cited references. Presenting a neat and attractive image is one of the least difficult ways to propose that you know how to organize your work. Writing in a clear, logically arranged sequence will make reviewing your proposal a pleasure. Making your figures, tables, and information easy to locate will gain you favor as well.

Using extraneous words quickly uses up your allowed space. Reduce the need to write lengthy paragraphs by using "bullets" or lists, tables, or figures. Avoid the temptation to put important details in the appendix, hoping the reviewers will seek it there. If it is important, state it briefly in the text of the proposal. In NIH reviews, the appendices are given only to the three or four main reviewers and not to the entire review committee.

Also use the numbered reference format instead of the author/year format for citing references. It is easy to see how a string of eight cited references might take an entire line of text, whereas a numbered reference format would simply list the range of numbers (e.g., 1–8). Using superscripts (as in the style of the *Journal of the American Medical Association*) saves space because the numbers are small and compact, which makes this style a favorite among NIH submissions. Be sure to check the accuracy of your references before grant submission because errors may be more common when making edits to text that have used the numbering format. Also remember to check for stipulations for using American Psychological Association (APA) format or other styles mentioned in your grant application guidelines.

* * *

SHOWING THAT YOU ARE A QUALIFIED APPLICANT

Your qualifications for carrying out a grant can be found in several places in your proposal. These include your (a) biographical sketch of education, experience, research, and publications; (b) preliminary studies section that explains your prior work relevant to the proposed grant; (c) letters of support and agreements; and (d) selection of collaborators. Holtzclaw in her "Six P's of Funding Qualifications" presents some general principles for demonstrating these qualifications to help you build this capacity (Holtzclaw, 2007). The list includes the following:

1. Program of research
2. Publications
3. Pilot or preliminary work
4. Previous funding support
5. Partners
6. Passion

Program of Research

A *program of research* shows that your proposed research "fits" with your previous history of scholarship (e.g., dissertation and/or thesis, pilot work, projects, courses, publications, future goals). Your future goals may be the most important item if you are a new graduate or if you are changing your area of interest. Not everyone who gets research funding fulfills each qualification, but the list is helpful in preparing for and writing the sections of your proposal that reveal your qualifications. This characteristic of your background assures grant reviewers that you not only are familiar with the proposed topic and/or methods, but also intend on developing it in the future. Developing a program of research lets you build on each succeeding step rather than going in many directions.

Publications

Publications are your retrievable milestones of research productivity and scholarship. They are included in your grant biographical sketch to give reviewers a quick indication of the types, topics, and numbers of publications you have produced. Scanning the dates of publication also reveals something about the consistency and continuity of your scholarly activity. Scanning the topics reveals how focused you have been.

Pilot or Preliminary Work

Pilot or preliminary work is included as a section in many grant application forms. This refers to *your* work and not to work found in the literature. Ideally, preliminary work includes findings that led you to the present study. This is a place where a program of research is highly beneficial in reflecting careful exploration of a topic, from small pilot work to more preliminary studies leading to the present proposal. If the proposed study is a pilot study and you have no preliminary work, include an explanatory statement (e.g., "there is no preliminary or pilot work," "the proposed study is the initial pilot for a future study of . . ."). Applicants sometimes include previous work on someone else's research study if they have gained expertise or experience with the methods or population related to the proposed study. The idea is to show how your previous research relates to the grant proposal.

Previous Funding Support

Previous funding support shows reviewers that you have successfully traveled this road before. You were entrusted with prior funding because you showed capability. It implies that you were able to manage these funds. The frosting on the cake is when you have a publication to show for each of your prior grants. A word of caution, however: Previous grants with no published findings raise a red flag of suspicion that funding has not yielded results.

Partners

Partners, meaning a research team and collaborators in research, are hallmarks of research capacity. Granted, research for your thesis or dissertation was probably a solitary activity. Beyond that, however, the ability to demonstrate that you have an established team of colleagues who offers expertise and commitment and collaborates on publications and previous research is a major strength in research qualifications. Partners also include community or agency partners granting you entrée to their facility, excellent consultation, and advisory committees to projects. For *community-engaged research* (see Chapter 6), the partnership is more than a hallmark of your success; it is the core of the proposal.

Passion

Passion for your topic and program of research is reflected in prior scholarship. Your work roles, community and professional contributions, prior research, and publications reflect your choices of topics and commitment. If they are consistent with the present proposal, it tells reviewers that the present topic is not a passing interest. Although you will not likely find *passion* on a grant reviewer's checklist, you will find statements evaluating your commitment to a particular research goal or topic.

• • •

ESTABLISHING THE NEED FOR YOUR PROPOSAL

Identifying the Need

Need is usually in the eye of the beholder, yet a successful grant application attempts to convince the funding agency that the statement of need expressed in the proposal is congruent with the agency's goals or missions. Perhaps your need for grant funding may be as simple as the need to evaluate and justify outcomes in a competitive managed healthcare environment. More commonly, however, grants are written for the purpose of funding one's own program of research and gaining release time from clinical or classroom teaching responsibilities for scholarly activities. Academicians often seek training grants to expand or significantly revise the curriculum within a college or university while keeping costs down by hiring program faculty specifically on the grant monies. This strategy allows the school to demonstrate the self-sufficiency and success of the program during the first 3 years (program grants are usually 3 to 5 years in length) before assuming the total costs involved in a new program. A special-projects or demonstration grant is sometimes used to facilitate the development of an educational or clinical program when no similar programs exist in a particular geographic area. Funds must often be obtained to demonstrate the efficacy of the program before the community will embrace the idea. For example, this strategy was used for the first school-based, nurse-run health clinics. Each of these situations reflects applicant-specific needs with aims that must be articulated in outcome-oriented language consistent with the funding organization's perception of need. Research needs must go beyond your own personal need to achieve tenure, complete a dissertation, or get published. The need your funding agency is interested in is why the *research*, not the funding, is necessary. The need should emerge clearly in the problem statement and the proposed study outcomes that address the need.

* * *

RECOGNIZING YOUR INVESTMENT IN THE PROCESS

The need for writing a grant may be a professional choice on your part, or the employing institution may dictate it. In either circumstance, writing a grant can often be very stressful. Having the self-determination and personal energy reserves necessary to survive the grueling parts of the grant writing process depends, in large part, on the commitment one has to the grant, the passion felt for the answer to the question, and the resources to assist in the process. One cannot and should not downplay the many sacrifices necessary to get a grant ready for a timely submission to an external funding agency. The sheer pressure of tight timelines and competing responsibilities of grant writing has turned many "angelic" Dr. Jekyll colleagues into grant writing "terrors" resembling Mr. Hyde. It is unpleasant to discover these hidden personalities when individuals turn unpleasant in the midst of the grant writing process. On the flip side are colleagues who thrive on the academic challenge of taking an idea and turning it into a fundable project. These colleagues form excellent collaborative teams that you will treasure and find helpful for present and future grant projects. Those finding themselves in the survival mode during the grant writing process are less likely to be successful in their efforts and certainly will make themselves, and perhaps others, miserable in the process. When not given a choice about writing the grant, the process becomes arduous, and the writer slips into survival mode. By contrast, the person approaching grant writing in the "thrival" mode views the future possibilities and opportunities provided by the experience; the potentially burdensome task of writing becomes an exciting intellectual adventure. The grant is the opportunity to answer that nagging clinical question or to develop a program or clinical project to meet an aggregate need. Not only is that personally exciting, but it also contributes to the body of scientific and theoretical knowledge.

This excitement overcomes the dread of the journey and creates the energy and focus needed to sustain the process of grant writing. The choice to survive or thrive in writing a grant is a personal one. Although jobs often depend on the task of grant writing, the individual has the option to view it as an arduous task or to be challenged about the opportunities and possibilities that the future holds for the successful grant writer.

● ● ●

FORMULATING A FUNDABLE IDEA

Developing a fundable idea takes ingenuity and skill in turning the idea into a meaningful question. Ideas may come from a number of sources, both clinically and professionally. Some of the best ideas often arise from clinical practice. This clinical base has been a rich resource of fundable research ideas. When Walden entered neonatal nursing in the late 1970s, healthcare professionals in the neonatal intensive care unit (NICU) did not believe that preterm infants had the autonomic or functional capacity to perceive pain because of their immature central nervous systems. Walden's clinical observations told her otherwise. After hearing the cries of infants during painful procedures, she questioned the current thinking about neonatal pain. This early professional observation was the source for her program of research and grant writing efforts. She could not, however, just go out and study neonatal pain. She needed equipment and personal resources. Writing a grant fit into her research plans.

Nursing-sensitive indicators or hospital-acquired conditions are excellent sources for generating clinical research questions. Aligning your research questions with organizational priorities are often win-win for both the researcher and the organization. Because patient-safety and quality-improvement initiatives are major focuses for healthcare organizations, these are major opportunities for improvement in science research and grant-funding opportunities. Clinical staff often need encouragement to transition their quality-improvement and evidence-based practice projects with insufficient evidence to formal research projects. Hospitals that employ nurse scientists offer great opportunities for assisting clinical staff in grant writing efforts to fund their clinically based research projects.

Regardless of the clinical area where one practices, evaluating the research base of that practice is a source of many fundable ideas. Gaps in the literature or conflicting results from previous studies provide another source of ideas for research and meaningful questions for a grant proposal. Questions that the literature leaves unresolved are great avenues for future research and, depending on the research priorities of the various funding agencies, are also great venues for external funding.

Professional conferences are other excellent sources for generating research ideas. One usually becomes energized at a conference and believes the world is conquerable. The power of networking with researchers in the field and talking with other healthcare professionals from around the country cannot be underestimated. Many researchers are anxious to replicate their studies in another setting or for their instruments to be retested. Both of these strategies add to their own database and research credibility. This replication provides novices a chance to use already developed and tested methods and data-collection instruments. Use of nationally known experts on grants as project team members or consultants increase the credibility of the grant application. Staying in touch with experts and engaging in conference networking allows one to become knowledgeable about what others are doing in a particular field, avoid duplicating current work, and avoid replicating errors. It allows the researcher to focus on a grant angle that has the potential for generating new knowledge or adding depth to existing knowledge. Furthermore, networking may also allow collaborative relationships to develop between individuals with similar interests. These interactions may help strengthen an idea or may lead to ideas not previously considered.

Identifying mentors in your topic area, whether for a research, training, or special-projects grants, has many advantages. Involving mentors not only allows the grant writer to use their expertise to develop the grant proposal, but also to set the stage for future collaborations. If these individuals are considered the experts in the field, they are likely to be scientists of the caliber the funding agency will use to review your proposal. Learning from the "master" as you shape your own ideas and educational or research program will be invaluable, as will the relationship you establish.

Although strong attention to literature and colleagues within your own area of interest may lead to a plausible grant idea, pushing the interdisciplinary envelope by exploring other related fields may produce novel ideas. Interdisciplinary research teams are encouraged and often lead to that novel approach to research. For example, Medoff-Cooper wished to study neurobehavioral development in preterm infants by observing their suck, swallow, and breathe coordination. Her collaboration with a biomedical engineer who developed a sucking device that would measure sucking pressure, amount of fluid delivered, and the suck-swallow-breathe patterns, led to a Small Business Innovative Research grant (Medoff-Cooper, McGrath, & Bilker, 2000). The device was useful in several other studies that followed and to other researchers needing to measure these variables.

Keeping abreast of advances in other fields can often give new insights into research questions. A still unanswered question about pain in neonates will likely be answered by molecular neurobiology. Parents of children who were preterm often report high pain thresholds in their infants. Researchers have found that changes in the infant's brain led to alterations in pain responses (Grunau, 2013). Now the research is focusing on neuroprotective factors in the NICU and beyond as knowledge of trauma-informed care has grown (Coughlin, 2016). Teams of researchers often include developmental specialists, nurses, physicians, physiologist, pain specialists, and others. Such observations, coupled with preliminary research findings, may stimulate the grant writer to draw on new and emerging concepts within the field of molecular neurobiology. These complex findings could offer plausible rationales for generating hypotheses for why these children have higher pain thresholds than healthy infants born at term. Subsequent studies could then explore and compare outcomes of effective interventions for minimizing the long-term effects of chronic, repeated pain in critically ill preterm infants. Along the same lines, journal clubs may be a source of ideas for future research questions. These meetings often point to differences in care practices between healthcare providers from different institutions. They may also lead to the realization that the current research base is insufficient to support a current therapeutic regimen and thus support the need for further research in this area.

• • •

MAKING ROOM FOR WRITING

Whatever the strategy you find helpful in generating ideas, it will be important to set aside time to think about all the information that you have gathered. One of the hindrances to the success of grant writers is busy schedules and other demands. In today's work setting, everyone is asked to work harder, often with fewer resources. By the end of the workday, you probably feel exhausted. Yet the work does not end there. Working at this level consistently promotes professional burnout and stifles creativity in grant writing. Successful grant writers and researchers often emphasize the need to selfishly protect sufficient time for scholarship. This dedicated time must fit your own work schedule and your knowledge of how you best function. One day a week or even a few hours each day are two variations of dedicated writing time. The schedule is up to you. You determine whatever works for you. Whatever it is, just do it!

Tips for Dedicating Time

Try the following tricks of the trade:

- If you find yourself spending too much time figuring out where you left off when writing in shorter work sessions, increase your productivity by scheduling longer sessions.
- If you spend too much time finding materials, reference books, prior drafts, or computer supplies before writing sessions, try creating a "portable office" by keeping these materials together in a briefcase, box, or suitcase.
- Determine what kind of environment increases your productivity. For some, it is a quiet environment free from distractions; for others, it might be the library.

• • •

ASKING THE RIGHT QUESTION

Determining whether yours is the "right question" involves considerable thought. Ideally, the right question is congruent with your own research interests. Your passion for the topic will help you persevere through the long, tedious grant writing process.

Your passion alone is not enough to gain research funding. It must also be of critical interest to others. The competitive nature of external funding requires that your area of interest be broad enough to appeal to a sufficient target population to warrant a grant award. This does not mean that you need to give up your original passion for a topic, but rather that you tailor your proposal to fit one of the funding priorities or initiatives available. Funding agencies often set broad research funding priorities, with many using *Healthy People 2020* objectives. On a global level, use the United Nations Sustainable Development Goals (2017), which are guiding healthcare changes. Some funding priorities are narrower, such as those dealing with a certain disease or symptom. You need to examine each of the potential funding agencies, determine their funding priorities, determine their individual rules for obtaining funds (such as using your professional association membership to access members-only funds or having certain credentials), and choose the best match for your particular area of interest.

While you consider targeting a specific priority or a broad focus, give your idea a unique slant. In fact, finding a novel or innovative angle to studying a problem is one of the areas that improve a grant reviewer's score. Often, the specific slant of your question needs to be tailored more directly to the funding priorities identified. For example, the National Institute of Nursing Research (NINR) has an ongoing call for proposals for health promotion among racial/ethnic minority males. The NINR goal of funding grants that develop and test culturally and linguistically appropriate health-promoting interventions designed to reduce health disparities among racially/ethnically diverse males is broad enough to accommodate a variety of specific questions and research approaches from individual and group studies to health-services research. Likewise, the initiative is broad enough to cover health behavioral studies as well as biologically based research.

CONCLUSION

Writing a great proposal starts with a great idea. Before starting to write any grant proposal, systematically review the literature, talk with experts in the field, and obtain consultations as necessary. Identify a question that is relevant, one that has the potential to generate new knowledge, solve a clinical management problem, or produce a new type of educational program. In addition, be sure your question is broad enough to be of interest to a significant portion of the funding source's population. By taking the time to do your homework and finding a match between your area of research and current funding options, you will substantially increase your success at obtaining grant monies.

REFERENCES

Boykova, M. (2016). Transition from hospital to home in preterm infants and their families. *Journal of Perinatal & Neonatal Nursing, 30*(3), 270–272. doi:10.1097/JPN.0000000000000198

Cohen, J. (1988). *Statistical power analysis for the behavioral sciences* (2nd ed.). Hillsdale, NJ: Erlbaum.

Cohen, J. (1990). Things I have learned (so far). *American Psychologist, 45*(12), 1304–1312. doi:10.1037/0003-066X.45.12.1304

Coughlin, M. E. (2016). *Trauma-informed care in the NICU: Evidenced-based practice guidelines for neonatal clinicians.* New York, NY: Springer Publishing. ISBN: 9780826131966

Dworkin, S. (2012). Sample size policy for qualitative studies using in-depth interviews. *Archives of Sexual Behavior, 41*(6), 1319–1320. doi:10.1007/s10508-012-0016-6

Grunau, R. E. (2013). Neonatal pain in very preterm infants: Long-term effects on brain, neurodevelopment and pain reactivity. *Rambam Maimonides Medical Journal, 4*(4), e0025. doi:10.5041/RMMJ.10132

Holtzclaw, B. J. (2007). *Characteristics of a fundable research grant.* Paper presented at the Second Research Conference of the Association of Nurses in AIDS Care, San Antonio, TX.

MacLean, P. S., Wing, R. R., Davidson, T., Epstein, L., Goodpaster, B., Hall, K. D., . . . Ryan, D. (2015). NIH working group report: Innovative research to improve maintenance of weight loss. *Obesity, 23*(1), 7–15. doi:10.1002/oby.20967

Medoff-Cooper, B., McGrath, J. M., & Bilker, W. (2000). Nutritive sucking and neurobehavioral development in preterm infants from 34 weeks PCA to term. *MCN, The American Journal of Maternal Child Nursing, 25*(2), 64–70.

National Institute of Mental Health. (2016). Letter of intent. Retrieved from https://www.nimh.nih.gov/funding/grant-writing-and-application-process/letter-of-intent.shtml

National Institutes of Health. (2018). How to apply—Application guide. Grants and funding. Retrieved from https://grants.nih.gov/grants/how-to-apply-application-guide.html

Sandelowski, M. (1995). Sample size in qualitative research. *Research in Nursing & Health, 18*(2), 179–183.

United Nations. (2017). Sustainable development goals: 17 goals to transform our world. Retrieved from http://www.un.org/sustainabledevelopment/sustainable-development-goals

3

. . .

What Type of Grant Do You Want?

. . .

IS YOUR IDEA A MATCH?

Many types of grants are available to healthcare professionals, but finding a match between your idea and the granting agency is an absolute necessity for funding success. Well-written proposals and superb ideas are unlikely be funded if an agency is not interested in the project. For this reason, you should always acquaint yourself with your funding source's goal and mission. If the match is possible, but not overtly obvious, then establishing the connection between your idea and the funding agency's goals becomes a priority in your grant proposal. If you are still unable to see a fit, move on! There are many more sources of funds.

. . .

HOW MUCH FUNDING DO YOU NEED?

Where you seek funding may be, in part, dictated by the amount of financial support your project needs. If you need "seed" money to support pilot work, a small conference, or a short-term survey, you may find a small grant sufficient. Foundations, practice and research organizations, universities, hospitals, institutions, and agencies are potential sources of small grants. Small grants are defined differently by different organizations, but they are typically under $50,000 and include no salary support. Very small seed grants may be as small as $100. Although the National Institutes of Health (NIH) sponsors a Small Grants Program (R03) that offers $50,000 per year for up to 2 years and includes salary support, this is not typical of small grants in general. NIH Small Grants are discussed under the section on federal funding.

Major or "large" grants, like smaller grants, are designated as such by those that award them. One typical feature that sets large grants apart is the support of salary, support personnel, major equipment, and institutional indirect costs. As in any grant submission choice, the decision to apply for a major grant should rest with your need and readiness to carry out a major project. Readiness for major funding, even for "new investigator" awards, generally involves some preliminary pilot work and evidence of capability. Some sources of grant funding are limited by geographic region, membership in a professional organization, place of employment, or career level. Primarily these grants fall into six categories: foundation grants, hospital-based or institutional grants, professional association grants, corporate partnerships, predoctoral and postdoctoral research training fellowships, and federal grants.

• • •

FOUNDATION GRANTS

Foundation grants are nongovernmental awards that support the mission and goals of specific philanthropic societies, corporate or organizational foundations, or charitable groups. According to the Foundation Center (n.d.), there are five types of foundations: independent, company sponsored, operating, community, and public charities. They may or may not have a specific funding cycle. Some foundations review grants when they are submitted. Others have timelines and guidelines for application. Certain health maintenance organizations, insurance companies, and managed care groups now have foundations that support community projects to increase the visibility of their organization. Professional association foundations, created to support their members, or company-sponsored foundations that support charitable causes are separate corporate entities from the parent organization. A professional association may require membership as a criterion for grant eligibility. Foundation grants may have a definite application deadline or a rolling deadline, which means that they review grants whenever one is received. Foundations sometime require a letter of intent, which describes the focus of the project in just a very few pages. It allows the foundation reviewers to determine whether the project is within the scope of the foundation's mission. If the project is acceptable to the mission, the grant seeker is asked to submit a full proposal according to specified guidelines. This "pre-proposal" offers an opportunity for the foundation to examine the match between your idea and their goals, as well as to gauge their interest in learning more about it. For the applicant, it saves the lengthy process of writing the full foundation proposal and waiting for the peer review. The foundation grant process is usually less intimidating and often provides a quicker turnaround time for an answer to whether or not the project is fundable. As a word of caution, the very brevity of a foundation grant can be a challenge. The human tendency is to give a lot of information instead of a concise presentation. Therefore, in many respects, short grants for a small award can require as much thought and careful editing than a lengthier grant for major funding. It is also wise to check with your organization before deciding to submit for a foundation grant. Many organizations attempt to prioritize submissions for foundation grants to eliminate internal competition and optimize their chance of receiving funding for a priority project.

Foundation grants are a nice way to start your attempts at funding. For most foundations, the submission process is fairly straightforward and brief compared with that for federal grants. They tend to provide small sums of money for very specific focus areas. These funds are excellent sources of seed money to start projects. For example, Kenner saw a call for proposals from the Purdue Frederick Foundation in a foundation's newsletter. Their areas of interest were perinatal healthcare. She submitted a brief proposal for a qualitative research study, "Transition from Hospital to Home for Mothers and Babies." The grant was awarded within 3 months of submission and was used to fund her dissertation. This seed money then gave her a good start to seek more funding for her next project that again focused on research on transitions. Holtzclaw needed a small grant to pilot her intervention study, "Control of Shaking Chills During Amphotericin B Therapy: A Pilot," during her postdoctoral work at the University of Pennsylvania. She submitted a proposal for an institutionally managed grant and was funded by the Mabel Pew Myrin Trust. This small award of $2,000 helped Holtzclaw to gain the preliminary evidence needed to launch a program of research and two major federally funded grant awards. The ability to successfully write a foundation grant gave her confidence that she could go on for other foundation monies as well as federal grants.

The March of Dimes Birth Defects Foundation of Greater Cincinnati awarded a larger grant to Kenner. She sought funds for a professional educational component of her Perinatal Alcohol Users grant funded by the Centers for Disease Control and Prevention (CDC). Foundation funds were to support an educational intervention aimed at increasing the awareness of health professionals about the harmful effect of perinatal alcohol use at any stage of pregnancy. As a clinician, she and other members of her research team felt they were seeing more women delivering alcohol-exposed babies in their prenatal clinics than the report rates reflected. The aim of the research to include health professional education about potential harmful birth defects from perinatal alcohol exposure fit with the March of Dimes Birth Defects Foundation's goals. The first step in the application process was a letter of intent to ensure there was a match between the project's specific aims and the foundation's mission. The March of Dime's Birth Defects Foundation's request for proposal was sent about 2 weeks following submission of their letter of intent. Kenner then submitted a full proposal. A positive funding decision arrived about 8 weeks after the proposal submission.

Kenner found other foundations helpful as her career developed. The University of Cincinnati Colleges of Medicine and Nursing sent a joint proposal to the Gates Foundation, requesting support for the education in medicine and nursing of faculty in Honduras. The proposed project was directed at providing faculty exchanges and eventually student exchanges. This was consistent with the Gates Foundation search for projects designed to increase the general educational level, not just that of health professionals, in developing countries. The application was very brief and required a concise synthesis of the project. Trimming the ideas down to a meaningful short version was more challenging than writing a longer proposal, although the process itself seemed less daunting.

The following are examples of foundations that provide grant opportunities:

- Alex's Lemonade Stand Foundation
- American Nurses Foundation
- American Organization of Nurse Executives Foundation for Nursing Leadership Research and Education
- Interact for Health (formerly ChoiceCare Foundation of Cincinnati, Ohio)
- Daisy Foundation
- Bill & Melinda Gates Foundation
- Gerber Foundation
- John A. Hartford Foundation
- Independent Blue Cross Foundation
- W. K. Kellogg Foundation
- March of Dimes Birth Defects Foundation
- David and Lucille Packard Foundation
- Pew Charitable Trusts Foundation
- RGK Foundation
- Robert Wood Johnson Foundation
- Rockefeller Foundation

These foundations change their focus or shift their priorities from time to time, so it is always best to consult their websites for current funding initiatives. Foundations that are associated with professional associations are discussed below.

A comprehensive resource on foundations, Foundation Center, is accessible at foundationcenter.org. Foundation Center was established in 1956 and supports more than 600 foundations. They are a leading authority on philanthropy with a mission to strengthen the nonprofit sector by advancing knowledge about U.S. philanthropy. Foundation Center maintains a comprehensive database on U.S. grant makers, provides several free search options, and makes their Foundation Directory Online available for a subscription fee.

• • •

HOSPITAL-BASED OR INSTITUTIONAL GRANTS

Hospitals, universities, school systems, and other institutions often offer grants that are generally offered only to employees of their organizations. The institution may request proposals for certain projects that they wish to see started. In the past, hospital or university grants were most likely to go to physicians or established scientists simply because other health professionals did not know they existed. These grants support small budgets, and they act as seed money for preliminary work or phases of an existing project. A wealthy donor may tie the funds to a specific type of research related to an institutional endowment. Other funds may be administered through a hospital foundation with the express purpose of furthering research that addresses a specific disease or enhances the healthcare of individuals served by the hospital.

A particularly positive aspect of partnering with a hospital is access to the patient population, especially if that is important in accomplishing the research. The clinical agency may have a need to provide sound clinical or quality improvement outcomes, but they may lack the available expertise or time to set up a research protocol. The emerging Magnet® hospitals have prompted considerable activity in both of these areas and may welcome your proposal and willingness to carry out their desired work. This is an excellent opportunity for academicians who may have the personal desire, as well as pressure from tenure and promotion committees, to do research but who lack access to the clinical setting. The "marriage" of the academic and clinical institutions can benefit both parties.

A good example of a local hospital-based grant came to the attention of Kenner's master's student in Cincinnati. The hospital sought to increase the customer satisfaction of their inpatient obstetric patients. Extending the previously mentioned research in "Transition from Hospital to Home for Mothers and Babies," the student wanted to do an extension of Kenner's transition research as her thesis. Professor and student approached a maternal/child clinical nurse specialist (CNS) who worked at an area level II nursery. The CNS was most anxious to make changes in the nursery's follow-up care for mothers and babies, but she needed evidence to support the need for more coordinated follow-up and teaching after discharge. She told of the funds her hospital provided for research. Within 2 months, the student wrote a proposal that served three purposes: extended Kenner's research to a new setting, gave her a master's thesis, and gave the CNS an opportunity to gain support for her clinical ideas. Another aspect of this process was that all of them were gaining experience in grant writing. The proposal was very short and easy to write. The project was funded in a few weeks. The master's student came out of the experience with a thesis and her first grant, and finished her study with a positive feeling toward research. For the hospital, the project provided the basis for what would eventually become a home follow-up program that netted a profit and good public relations.

• • •

PROFESSIONAL ASSOCIATION GRANTS

Many professional associations offer grant opportunities to their members. These grants are administered either directly by the association or through an auxiliary foundation. Corporate sponsors of the association sometimes partner with the professional society to offer educational scholarships or research grants. For example, equipment companies that exhibit their wares at healthcare conferences also allocate monies to an association for the express purpose of a research protocol that tests their equipment. This type of grant would be a focused or targeted grant. Practice-focused associations, such as the Oncology Nurses Society (ONS), have associated foundations that give seed monies once per year to grantees who want to conduct research in the areas targeted by the association. Foundation grants linked with nursing specialty associations generally support research in the area of specialty focus. As the nursing shortage has increased, so has the number of scholarships or foundation grants that are aimed at education. Educational endeavors are aimed at increasing the level of education of nurses in the specialty focus. A benefit to the foundation is that such grants attract members to their parent association. Organizational research grant recipients are often required to present their research findings at the organization's national or regional conference. Membership in the association is usually a prerequisite to the application process.

The American Nurses Foundation (ANF) is the philanthropic arm of the American Nurses Association and a good example of a foundation that supports research and special projects across nursing specialties. The foundation awards a number of small research grants ranging from $3,500 to $25,000 to beginning and experienced nurse researchers. Some ANF grants are generated internally by ANF endowment funds, whereas others receive annual external support from contributions to the ANF Nursing Research Grants Program by nursing organizations such as Sigma Theta Tau International, the regional research groups (e.g., Western Institute of Nursing, Midwest Nursing Research Society, Southern Nursing Research Society, Eastern Research Nursing Association), and the Council for the Advancement of Nursing Science. Other external contributions come from ANA'S Presidential Scholar Fund, the Commissions on Graduates of Foreign Nursing Schools, and corporate foundations. Because some of the funding streams for ANF grants vary each year, applicants should examine closely the availability, eligibility, and level of funding for these grants in the specific year they wish to apply. Although ANA membership is not required for applying for ANF grants, those sponsored by nursing organizations and regional research groups are required to have membership in their specific group. Several of the ANF grants are specifically targeted at a special topic or individuals with a designated level of preparation, whereas others are without restrictions. Two surveys of ANF research grant recipients over its 60-year history demonstrate the long-range impact on nursing science made by these small grants (Holtzclaw, 2006; Messmer, Zalon, & Phillips, 2014). Recipients include many of today's top nurse scientists who credited the initial boost of their program of research to the ANF funding of their pilot work.

Professional association grants represent nearly every nursing specialty, and many are distributed directly from the association itself. The following are just a few examples:

- Society of Pediatric Nurses (SPN) awards a $1,000 Corrine Barnes Nursing Research Grant.
- International Society of Nurses in Genetics (ISONG) Nursing Research Small Grant Program supports research related to genetic nursing practice or practice that contributes to the development of genetic nursing science.
- American Cancer Society Targeted Grants for Research Directed at Poor and Underserved Populations is designed to support research that addresses the disparity in cancer morbidity and mortality in poor and underserved populations. This initiative includes research that addresses a variety of clinical, cancer control, behavioral, epidemiologic, health policy, health services, and basic science questions.
- The Oncology Nursing Society (ONS) Foundation provides three types of research grants that include education support, career development, or special topic support for specialized training in transplantation or end-of-life care, dissertation, or capstone project support.
- The American Association of Critical-Care Nurses (AACN) offers a variety of grants for research that is relevant to acute critical care nursing practice.
- The National Association of Pediatric Nurse Associates and Practitioners (NAPNAP) Foundation offers grants for nursing research that contributes to the improvement of quality of life for children and their families.
- The Association of Perioperative Registered Nurses supports the development of nurse researchers to contribute to the scientific knowledge related to perioperative nursing practice.
- NAPNAP Graduate Student Research Award was developed to support child and family research among graduate students.
- American Association of Colleges of Nursing supports educational grants that focus on programs, scholarships, or research.

- National League for Nurses supports educational research grants that are aligned with the organization's mission.
- American Public Health Association funds, for example, grants that examine maternal child health issues.

• • •

CORPORATE PARTNERSHIPS

Corporate partnerships often award grants for research, product development, implementation, or evaluation. These partnerships or strategic alliances are forged directly with a researcher/educator, an academic institution, or a professional association. These grants are viewed with skepticism by some professionals out of concern that researchers might be pressured to change study findings or not report them if they do not support the company's view. Although there is always an element of pressure from companies seeking to disassociate their "good name" from negative press, the responsibility rests with the researcher or grant seeker to clearly investigate the parameters of data ownership before signing on the bottom line. Among the information needed are the steps that must be followed for reporting, presenting, and publishing the data. In other words, who owns the data and who has the right to manipulate it? These are important up-front questions that must be answered before any partnerships are forged.

A researcher exploring funding support for a certain type of equipment or protocol that is to be used may seek corporate partnership grants from companies that produce these products. Seeking support from that company can make good sense for this type of partnership and can be a win-win arrangement for both parties as long as each party is clear about the expectations of the research and the dissemination of the findings. If a researcher is interested in this type of relationship, then either the local sales representative for the company or the research and development department of the company is an appropriate contact. Many larger companies have at least one person, if not a whole department of people, responsible for clinical research. Some even have "loan closets" from which small devices and equipment may be borrowed by responsible researchers. Often, the researcher can help the company gain entry to a clinical or academic setting that otherwise would be closed to them. The researcher should remember to check with their organization's legal or research-compliance officer before entering into an industry-sponsored research study. Contracts require negotiation for items such as salary support for data collectors, data ownership and publication rights, and institutional review board review costs. Corporate grants can open possibilities to do international, multisite studies that in the past were difficult to perform unless the researcher had the right connections. Today, with the globalization of industry, the corporate world provides opportunities to use already-established markets for their products as research sites.

Examples of corporate partnership grants include the following:

- AbbVie funds research regarding pharmacologic intervention with respiratory syncytial virus.
- Roche U.S. Pharmaceuticals funds studies based on genomics (study of encoded information in DNA) that examines the sequence of infectious pathogens and drugs to combat them.
- Novo Nordisk funds community-based projects, for example, that address ways to combat childhood obesity and type 2 diabetes.
- Janssen Biotech, Inc., funds scholarships and simulation.
- C. R. Bard, Inc., funds scholarships.

● ● ●

FELLOWSHIPS FOR PREDOCTORAL AND POSTDOCTORAL RESEARCH TRAINING

Predoctoral and postdoctoral fellowships are expressly for career development and training of professionals interested in specializing in a focused area of research or education. Most of these fellowships support part, if not all, the academic costs associated with moving into a higher level of education or research sophistication. Foundations, associations, or the federal government offer these grants.

A *predoctoral fellowship* focuses on gaining further education and training for a person who has not attained a doctoral degree but who is committed to seek further research and education. These fellowships pay for tuition and a stipend for the grantee's doctoral education. Most predoctoral fellowships include research training and experience with mentors to give the professional a new skill set to conduct research and apply competitively for research grants. It is one way that academic institutions can groom professionals for academic life that includes an active research career.

Postdoctoral grants are aimed at perfecting and honing already existing research skills. Generally, grants in these highly specialized areas of expertise are offered for 1 to 2 years of in-depth studies. Today, many are focused on laboratory or clinical science research in the areas of pain, the human genome, and cancer treatments. Other hot topics are ethics, workplace analysis, health policy, precision medicine or health, and interdisciplinary research programs.

The purpose of predoctoral and postdoctoral fellowships is to create a cadre of scholars across disciplines that will lead the health profession into the future. The rapid growth of technology has made it essential to have experts who can set the direction and give vision to the profession. Predoctoral training is designed to move the postbaccalaureate scholar toward the doctorate. Many doctoral programs in nursing with significant NIH funding are recruiting BSN graduates to their doctoral program trajectory. Postdoctoral scholars are defined by the NIH and the National Science Foundation as "an individual who has received a doctoral degree (or equivalent) and is engaged in a temporary and defined period of mentored advanced training to enhance the professional skills and research independence needed to pursue his or her chosen career path." Excellent tips for applying for NIH National Research Service Award (NRSA) fellowship grants were provided in an article by Parker and Steeves (2005), and information is provided online by NIH for specific NRSA awards (National Institute on Deafness and Other Communication Disorders, 2016). The two types of NRSA awards are Institutional (T) and Individual (F) training awards. NRSA Institutional training grants are awarded by the NIH to universities or institutions with specific training foci (e.g., genomics, neurosciences, end-of-life, chronic illness). Because these grants are only given for a specified time, you must look at what T awards are currently being funded to an institution (www .nigms.nih.gov/training/pages/InstGrantLists.aspx). You must apply for these awards directly to the institution, and information will be provided by the university to which you apply. A research proposal must be well fleshed out and reflect the prerequisite or planned coursework to support the proposed research. NRSA Individual Predoctoral and Postdoctoral awards require the applicant to have a pre-existing cooperative agreement with a mentor who has major funding. Because the scholarship awards only tuition and a stipend to the student, the application must reflect the mentor's commitment and ability to support the academic expertise, guidance, and provision of laboratory equipment, supplies, and research resources. Both types of NRSA programs encourage awardees to seek pilot funding while they are NRSA fellows. This not only helps support their project costs, but also helps develop grantsmanship skills.

Examples of NRSA and Foundation predoctoral and postdoctoral fellowship grants include the following:

- Pfizer Postdoctoral Fellowship Program
- NRSA Training Grants and Fellowships that include the following:
  - Ruth L. Kirschstein NRSA Institutional Predoctoral Fellowships (T32) are awarded to university units with a significant number of existing federally funded studies in a focused topic area (topics vary from palliative care to biobehavioral research). Students are usually funded 2 to 3 years.
  - Ruth L. Kirschstein NRSA Individual Predoctoral Fellowships (F31) are awarded to individuals submitting high-quality proposals and demonstrating a match with significantly funded research mentors in institutions with suitable resources to support the work.

- NRSA Individual Postdoctoral (F32) Fellowships are awarded to individuals seeking a defined period of mentored advanced training who submit high-quality proposals and demonstrate a match with significantly funded research mentors in institutions with suitable resources to further the applicant's previous work. Students are usually funded 2 to 4 years.
- NIH NRSA Individual Predoctoral Fellowships for Minority Students (F31) provide up to 5 years of support for research training leading to the doctorate. Fellowships are designed to enhance the racial/ethnic diversity of the biomedical, behavioral, and health services research labor force in the United States.
- NIH NRSA Predoctoral Fellowships for Students with Disabilities (F31) provide up to 5 years of support for research training leading to the doctorate and are designed to encourage students with disabilities to seek graduate degrees and increase the number of scientists with disabilities prepared to pursue careers in biomedical and behavioral research.

* * *

FEDERAL GRANTS

Federal funding offers some of the largest grants and best administered research funding in the nation. Much of the funding for healthcare is administered through the U.S. Department of Health and Human Services (USDHHS), which oversees the following U.S. Public Health Service (USPHS) agencies:

- NIH
- Agency for Healthcare Research and Quality (AHRQ)
- CDC
- Indian Health Services (IHS)
- Bureau of Health Workforce (BHW)

Federal Mechanisms and Codes

Different levels of federal funding are categorized by a *funding mechanism*. Familiarizing yourself with the various funding mechanisms and codes assigned to each will make it easier to locate grants that are appropriate for your experience and interests. Each NIH funding mechanism is designated with a three-digit code consisting of a letter and number (e.g., F32, K12, P01, R01, T32). The letters preceding the mechanism code indicate the general category of the grant and include:

- F—Fellowships
- K—Career development awards
- N—Research contracts
- P—Program project and research center grants
- R—Research project grants
- S—Research-related programs
- T—Training grants
- U—Cooperative agreements
- Y—Interagency agreements

The numbers that follow indicate the activity code and are specific to the level of funding and activity to which the award can be made. Research mechanisms most commonly used by the National Institute of Nursing Research (NINR) include the following:

R 01   **Research Project:** To support a discrete, specified, circumscribed project to be performed by named investigators in areas representing their specific interest and competencies.

R 03   **Small Research Grant:** To provide research support specifically limited in time and amount for studies in categorical program areas. Small grants provide flexibility for initiating studies that are generally for preliminary short-term projects and are nonrenewable.

R 15   **Academic Research Enhancement Awards (AREA):** To support small research projects conducted by faculty in domestic institutions awarding primarily baccalaureate degrees.

R 21   **Exploratory/Developmental Grants:** To encourage the development of new research activities in categorical program areas (generally restricted in level of support and time).

R 25   **Education Program Grants:** To support the development and implementation of curriculum-dependent programs that focus on educational activities before, during, or after the completion of a terminal doctoral degree. They must address a need that is not funded by another NIH mechanism.

K 01   **Research Scientist Development Award—Research and Training:** To support a scientist, committed to research, in need of both advanced research training and additional experience. Other K awards (e.g., K02, K05, K06, ranging to K99) are designed for advanced levels of research, training, and/or mentorship and have specific targeted activities assigned to each.

K 02 **Research Scientist Development Award—Research:** To support a scientist who is committed to research and in need of additional experience.

New mechanisms and activity codes continue to evolve in NIH funding. For this reason, it is important to use the latest updated information from the NIH web site at www.nih.gov when selecting a mechanism.

National Institutes of Health

The NIH began as a laboratory for hygiene in 1887. It has grown into 27 separate institutes and centers. The mission is to uncover new knowledge for the betterment of health. It is one of the eight health agencies under the USPHS, a part of the USDHHS. The NIH sets research priorities in each of the institutes and publicizes them on its website. Approximately 10% of research dollars goes to intramural research programs; the remainder goes toward extramural research. The intramural projects are conducted within the confines of the NIH campus, and extramural projects can be anywhere in the world. The current institutes and centers are as follows:

- National Cancer Institute
- National Eye Institute (NEI)
- National Heart, Lung, and Blood Institute
- National Human Genome Research Institute
- National Institute on Aging (NIA)
- National Institute on Alcohol Abuse and Alcoholism (NIAAA)
- National Institute of Allergy and Infectious Diseases (NIAID)
- National Institute of Arthritis and Musculoskeletal and Skin Diseases (NIAMS)
- National Institute of Biomedical Imaging and Bioengineering (NIBIB)
- Eunice Kennedy Shriver National Institute of Child Health and Human Development (NICHD)
- National Institute on Deafness and Other Communication Disorders (NIDCD)
- National Institute of Dental and Craniofacial Research (NIDCR)
- National Institute of Diabetes and Digestive and Kidney Diseases (NIDDK)
- National Institute on Drug Abuse (NIDA)
- National Institute of Environmental Health Sciences (NIEHS)
- National Institute of General Medical Sciences (NIGMS)
- National Institute of Mental Health (NIMH)
- National Institute on Minority Health and Health Disparities (NIMHD)
- National Institute of Neurological Disorders and Stroke (NINDS)

- NINR
- National Library of Medicine (NLM)
- Center for Information Technology (CIT)
- Center for Scientific Review (CSR)
- Fogarty International Center (FIC)
- National Center for Advancing Translational Science (NCATS)
- National Center for Complementary and Integrative Health (NCCIH)
- Clinical Center (CC)

The NIH funds health professionals and scientists across disciplines. Most grants are competitive, and the requests for proposals or applications are available through their website (www.nih.gov). The dates or cycles of funding, as well as the priorities, are listed. The main source of information is through the NIH Guide to Grants and Contracts. The contact person at the NIH is included in all postings about grants, and it is this person's job to assist with grant preparation. Use their expertise. Remember, the contact person is there to help potential grantees submit the best possible grant. All NIH agencies (including NINR, CDC, USDHHS, and AHRQ) use similar application processes and the PHS-398 form unless otherwise specified.

National Institute of Nursing Research

The NINR is only one of the NIH institutes. It is discussed separately because many nurses apply for its grant monies. In 1985, the NINR was first established as the National Center for Nursing Research. In 1986, the center moved under the auspices of NIH. Finally, in 1993 the Center was changed to an Institute, opening a portion of the NIH funds to its services. The structure and function of NINR changed: Becoming an institute gave it an equal status with the other institutes of health. Fund allocations now came from the general NIH budget. This placed nursing research (even though non-nurses can apply) on par with other disciplines at a federal level.

The National Advisory Council for Nursing Research, composed primarily of nurses, provides a second-level review of grants. The Council recommends to the director of the NINR which grants should be funded. Each grant that is submitted receives a priority score, but only a certain percentage is awarded funding. The grants are judged on scientific merit and the relevance of the proposed project to the NINR'S funding priorities.

The NINR also supports the training of nurse researchers for expanding the cadre of nurse researchers, and current budget requests include a 2% increase for stipend levels. The NINR also funds career-development grants and core centers in specialized areas of research. A portion of the NINR funding goes toward intramural programs; the remaining funds are used for extramural research programs. The NINR participates in joint research programs with the USDHHS, the Health Resources & Services Agency (HRSA), AHRQ, and the CDC.

The mission of NINR is to promote and improve the health and quality of life of individuals, families, and communities. For recent information on NINR'S Strategic Plan, please see the published statement "Advancing Science, Improving Lives: NINR'S new Strategic Plan and the Future of Nursing Science" (Grady, 2017). There is a strong emphasis on clinical research involving direct patient contact or basic science linked directly to patient problems. Current NINR funding priorities are consistent with those of NIH and include the following:

- Big Data to Knowledge
- Epigenetics
- Genetic Basis for Childhood Cancers and Structural Birth Defects
- Health Care Systems Research
- Symptom Science: Promoting Personalized Medicine
- Wellness: Promoting Health and Preventing Disease
- Self-Management: Improving Quality of Life for Individuals with Chronic Illness
- End-of-Life and Palliative Care: The Science of Compassion
- 21st-Century Nurse Scientists: Innovative Strategies for Research Careers
- Promoting Innovation: Technology to Improve Health

Centers for Disease Control and Prevention

The CDC is one of the major operating mechanisms of the USDHHS. The CDC'S mission is to promote health and the quality of life by the control and prevention of disease, injury, and disability. CDC'S strategic priorities are threefold: (a) to improve health security at home and around the world; (b) to better prevent the leading causes of illness, injury disability, and death; and (c) to strengthen public health and healthcare collaboration. The CDC includes 24 centers, institutes, and offices, including the following:

- Center for Global Health
- National Institute for Occupational Safety and Health
- Office of Infectious Diseases
- National Center for Emerging and Zoonotic Infectious Diseases
- National Center for HIV/AIDS, Viral Hepatitis, STD, and TB Prevention

- National Center for Immunization and Respiratory Diseases
- Office of Noncommunicable Diseases, Injury and Environmental Health
- National Center on Birth Defects and Developmental Disabilities
- National Center for Chronic Disease Prevention and Health Promotion
- National Center for Environmental Health
- National Center for Injury Prevention and Control
- Office of Public Health Preparedness and Response
- Office of Public Health Scientific Services
- National Center for Health Statistics
- Center for Surveillance, Epidemiology and Laboratory Services
- Office for State, Tribal, Local, and Territorial Support

The CDC does not fund individuals, but awards and administers grants and cooperative agreements to state and local governments, foreign ministries and associations, domestic nonprofits/educational institutions, and domestic for-profit groups.

USDHHS Training Grants

The USDHHS is the largest grant funding agency in the federal government. The department contains the following:

- Administration for Children and Families (ACF)
- Administration for Community Living (ACL)
- AHRQ
- Agency for Toxic Substances and Disease Registry (ATSDR)
- CDC
- Centers for Medicare & Medicaid Services (CMS)
- Food and Drug Administration (FDA)
- HRSA
- IHS
- NIH
- Substance Abuse and Mental Health Services Administration (SAMHSA)

The mission is to enhance the health and well-being of Americans through support of effective health and human services and by fostering sound, sustained advances in the sciences underlying medicine, public health, and social services. The USDHHS strategic goals focus on strengthening healthcare, advancing scientific knowledge and innovation, and advancing the health, safety, and well-being of the American people and improving quality of care through health services and education. One of the core values is to form partnerships with government, universities, and the private sector to improve quality of care. The USDHHS challenges that affect quality of care follow:

- Managed care transformation
- Rising number of uninsured Americans
- Changes in the composition of the American family
- Aging of America
- Rising costs associated with chronic illness
- Need for collaborative healthcare partnerships; patients' need for care coordination among specialists attending their health needs
- Genetic breakthroughs
- Threats of bioterrorism
- Privacy of healthcare information
- Emerging and re-emerging infectious diseases
- Changing role of the government in healthcare (USDHHS, 2004)

The USDHHS is the largest grant making agency in the United States. To submit a USDHHS grant, you must first register with the Data Universal Numbering System (D-U-N-S), System for Award Management (SAM), and Grants.gov. Grant making agencies and associated information can be found at www.grants.gov/web/grants/learn-grants/grant-making-agencies.html.

The USDHHS provides funding opportunities for educational grants. Some are very specific to a disease entity such as cancer education, whereas others are for basic or advanced education. Beginning in fiscal year 2000, Advanced Education Nursing Traineeship Grants that were previously funded require recipients to reapply. Only one grant application from an institution is recommended for grants that are similar in content. For example, a primary care women's health nurse practitioner grant and a pediatric nurse practitioner training grant from the same institution could be combined to simplify panel review and allow each grant to compete against one another. If the grants, however, are from different areas or there is a compelling need for each grant, then the institution may choose to submit more than one grant during a funding cycle. These changes are part of the Nursing Education and Practice Improvement Act of 1998.

Training grants are well known to most educators. They provide the monies to support nursing programs, especially at the advanced practice level. These grants are part of Title VIII of the Public Health Service Act, programs administered by the HRSA, Bureau of Health Professions, Division of Nursing. The purpose of these grants is to support education with the long-term outcome of improving healthcare delivery. The funding cycle is generally once or twice per year but depends on the grant. Grants are reviewed on the merits of the curriculum, availability of faculty, faculty expertise and credentials, and media resources, as well as the potential to draw a population of students. The request for proposals or applications can be found with other federal grants at the HRSA website (www.hrsa.gov/grants/fundingopportunities/default.aspx).

Examples of these training grants are numerous and include the following:

- Academic Administrative Units in Primary Care
- Predoctoral Training in Primary Care
- Physician Assistants Training in Primary Care
- Residency Training in Primary Care
- Faculty Development in Primary Care
- Podiatric Residency in Primary Care
- Model State-Supported Area Health Education Center (AHEC)
- Geriatric Education Centers
- Geriatric Training Regarding Physicians and Dentists
- Allied Health Special Projects, Public Health Training Centers
- Health Administration Traineeships and Special Projects
- Health Careers Opportunity Program
- Centers of Excellence
- Basic Nurse Education and Practice
- Advanced Education Nursing
- Nursing Workforce Diversity
- Advanced Education Nursing Traineeships
- Advanced Education Nursing—Nurse Anesthetist Traineeships
- Public Health Experience in State and Local Health Departments for Baccalaureate Nursing Programs

During this time of a critical nursing shortage, training grants are an important aspect of recruitment and retention of faculty positions. Undergraduate and graduate student enrollments have significantly dropped over the last 5 years. The USDHHS has funds available to schools that are interested in recruiting minority students and faculty and then retaining them. The USDHHS places a high priority in getting junior high and high school students excited about a health services career. Thus, a part of the undergraduate or special-projects grants contain an element of Kids Into Health Careers, a program aimed at marketing the positive aspects of health careers. Schools must include how they are going to implement this form of marketing. A major debate has arisen over the past few years about whether the training grant is able to demonstrate retention and strong recruitment strategies. Recruitment costs are high and not profitable to the nursing profession if they are not successful in retaining students.

Training grants at the advanced practice level are more likely to have a community-based focus and some component of distance learning. Some grants have demonstrated the need for a specific specialty program within a geographic area. The institutions, however, may lack the faculty expertise or dollars to support a freestanding program. For example, the University of Kansas, University of Missouri, and Wichita State University formed a consortium program for neonatal nurse practitioners, and the University of Cincinnati College of Nursing and Ohio State University started a joint nurse midwifery program. The latter was funded at the state, rather than federal, level. In each of these examples, the partnership meant bringing together competitors to sit at the table and work out a joint curriculum; if this hadn't happened, neither program would be able to start. Are these joint programs difficult? Yes, at times, but it is a successful strategy for receiving federal funds.

Many schools also recognize that at the graduate level they cannot be all things to all people; thus, centers of excellence are being established. An institution builds a reputation for a certain type of graduate education such as oncology nursing or substance abuse. The center concept provides a strong support component for resources when other grant funds for specific education are sought. Center grants are also available through various governmental agencies. Center grant writing is beyond the scope of this chapter, but it is important to remember that they exist and remain a potential source of funding in certain well-established research academic or healthcare centers. The Center Training Grant may provide a tangible commitment on the part of the institution to support specific, focused training.

Agency for Healthcare Research and Quality

The AHRQ was founded in 1989 to bridge the gap between biomedical research knowledge and the delivery of health care. A few of the past areas of focus have included Project ECHO (Extension for Community Healthcare Outcomes), Re-Engineered Discharge (RED), the Comprehensive Unit-based Safety Program (CUSP), EvidenceNOW, and TeamSTEPPS. This agency supports both intramural and extramural research. The current priorities are to (a) improve health care quality by accelerating implementation of patient-centered outcomes research (PCOR), (b) make health care safer, (c) increase accessibility by evaluating expansions of insurance coverage, and (d) improve healthcare affordability, efficiency, and cost transparency (AHRQ, 2012). Areas that the AHRQ is focusing on to make healthcare safer and better tomorrow include (a) reducing antibiotic overuse and eliminating healthcare-associated infections, (b) improving care for people with chronic conditions, (c) incorporating the latest research findings into electronic health records to facilitate clinical decision making, and (d) discovering how to better provide opioid addiction treatment services in rural communities. Extramural research may be supported through grant applications or cooperative agreements and contracts. Requests for proposals or applications are available at the AHRQ web site (www.ahrq .gov/funding/policies/foaguidance/index.html). The time cycle is included in the information found at this site.

Some grants are given only annually, whereas others are rolling (submission is not time dependent). Project officers are ready and willing to help the potential grantee write a successful grant. They encourage calls early in the grant writing process. The AHRQ suggests that a 3- to-7-page concept paper be submitted first for critique rather than waiting to submit an entire grant. This concept paper is not required. Grants are reviewed for scientific and technical merit and how well they fit with the priorities of the agency. This agency looks at grants as to their policy relevance or impact on policy making. Use of an interdisciplinary team is favored in research grants. A population or aggregate focus is also suggested. It is not uncommon for the project officer to contact the principal investigator once the initial review is completed. This call usually is to clarify certain aspects of the grant, including institutional capacity to carry it out. This practice is generally not done by other federal agencies. As with the other federal agencies, the AHRQ funds R01 (research grants that meet priority areas), R03 (small grants, which are often pilots or dissertation grants), R13 (conference grants), and F32 grants (individual postdoctoral research training grants).

Corporate or Small Business Grants

Corporate or small business grants may be awarded by specific corporations or foundations, as well as through the small business grant office at the federal level, primarily through the Office of Extramural Research of the NIH. The NIH offers Small Business Innovation Research (SBIR) grants and Small Business Technology Transfer (STTR) grants.

The SBIR program's aim is to support small businesses that have the potential for commercializing research. Biomedical and behavioral research are two of the priority funding areas. The STTR program is a cooperative agreement between a small business and a research institution. Innovation and commercialization of research are two of the major criteria for these grants. On the website (www .grants.nih.gov/grants/funding/sbir.htm) there is a link to the previous SBIR and STTR awards, which provides an abstract of successful grants and contact information on the project directors.

Funding is also available from venture capitalists who are independent contractors or associated with larger parent companies. For venture capitalists, the return may be a percentage of the business or they may offer to buy the company if it supports other corporations that they own. The list of potential companies is endless. There are online services such as Federal Money Retriever that will match a business with a potential financial backer. State departments of commerce are another good resource. For example, the state of Illinois has an initiative to advance Illinois technology. Funds are available to support science and technology projects, university commercialization centers, and technology transfer activities. Other resources are universities themselves; West Texas A&M University, University of Cincinnati, and Indiana University have all supported special projects, including small businesses.

Recently, small business grants have emphasized start-up monies for women attempting to start their own businesses. These businesses can be for-profit or not-for-profit companies. The grant applications are clear about what is or is not be covered. Like all other grants, the funding priorities are available.

Examples of resources for small business grants beside those listed include professional organizations and magazines. They include *Entrepreneur Magazine*, National Association for Female Executives, National Association of Women Business Owners, and Service Corps of Retired Executives (SCORE).

Special Projects of Regional and National Significance

Special Projects of Regional and National Significance (SPRANS) grants are special projects or demonstration programs that are funded through the Maternal Child Health Bureau (MCHB) and other federal agencies such as the HRSA. The thrust is to support innovative programs, training, and research in maternal and child health. For example, the Cincinnati Center for Developmental Disorders and Children's Hospital Adolescent Clinic identified a need for more training in adolescent health issues for physicians and nurses. The director of nursing at the adolescent clinic spearheaded the writing of several SPRANS grants to support educational activities. A few of these SPRANS projects evolved into nursing electives for the University of Cincinnati's undergraduate and graduate students. Traineeships for health professionals that desired training in adolescent health were also made available through SPRANS support. These cooperative agreements focus on health insurance and financing for children (FederalGrants .com, n.d.).

Demonstration projects highlight changes in healthcare delivery or in the community's healthcare needs. The rationale for these programs is to determine the feasibility of providing a service or expanding an educational program such as adolescent health education. If the pilot project is successful, other funding sources or the parent organization, such as a university, takes over the continuing costs. These projects generally provide strong positive public relations for the institution because they serve a community need. These grants can be a win-win situation. The downside is that when the funding dries up, these programs end, returning a population of patients to having no services again. This situation has happened many times when substance abuse clinics have been started, run well for the funding cycle, and then closed once the funds were gone. Reassurances are supposed to be made to the funding source that programs will continue at least for a time after the project's end, but in these tight financial times that is not always possible.

Another example is Georgetown University's National Center for Education in Maternal and Child Health. This program represents a SPRANS Synthesis Project to bring together information and data derived from SPRANS programs across the country. These data are used to support needs for other grants or to change practice services. Healthy Tomorrows Partnership for Children Program (HTPCP) Analysis and Synthesis Project–Georgetown University is an example of a grant that is impacting practice. This project includes support from the American Academy of Pediatrics to blend public health resources with professional pediatric expertise. The synthesis aspect of this program includes data from 107 nationwide projects. These are but two examples of special projects. The website, www.ncemch.org/projects.php, provides links to other projects.

CONCLUSION

Many resources exist for funding. Some of these monies are awarded only for research, whereas others are for educational and demonstration projects. The latter grant category helps support new, innovative clinical programs or expansion of existing programs to meet community healthcare needs. The entrepreneur also has resources within the federal government and private sector to "grow" a small business. These small businesses provide services to healthcare professionals or their patients that otherwise might not be available.

REFERENCES

Agency for Healthcare and Research and Quality. (2012). Funding opportunity announcement (FOA) guidance. Retrieved from https://www.ahrq.gov/funding/policies/foaguidance/index.html

FederalGrants.com. (n.d.). SPRANS cooperative agreement programs: Health insurance & financing for children with special health. Retrieved from http://www.federalgrants.com/SPRANS-Cooperative-Agreement-Programs-Health-Insurance-Financing-for-Children-with-Special-Health-17582.html

Foundation Center. (n.d.). Foundation grants to individuals online. Retrieved from foundationcenter.org/products/foundation-grants-to-individuals-online

Grady, P. A. (2017). Advancing science, improving lives: NINR's new strategic plan and the future of nursing science. *Journal of Nursing Scholarship, 49*(3), 247–248. doi:10.1111/jnu.12286

Holtzclaw, B. J. (2006). In good company: Celebrating 50 years of American Nurses Foundation research scholars. *Nursing Outlook, 54*(1), 17–22. doi:10.1016/j.outlook.2005.09.009

Messmer, P. R., Zalon, M. L., & Phillips, C. (2014). ANF scholars (1955–2012): Stepping stones to a nursing research career. *Applied Nursing Research, 27*(1), 2–24. doi:10.1016/j.apnr.2013.10.009

National Institute on Deafness and Other Communication Disorders. (2016). National Research Service Awards. Retrieved from https://www.nidcd.nih.gov/training/fellowship-awards

Parker, B., & Steeves, R. (2005). The National Research Service Award: Strategies for developing a successful proposal. *Journal of Professional Nursing, 21*(1), 23–31. doi:10.1016/j.profnurs.2004.11.009

U.S. Department of Health and Human Services. (2004). FY 2004 budget in brief. Retrieved from http://wayback.archive-it.org/3920/20130927185843/http://archive.hhs.gov/budget/04budget/fy2004bib.pdf

4

· · ·

It Takes a Village (and the Village Has a System!)

· · ·

GRANT WRITING IS NOT A SOLO SPORT

Writing a grant cannot be effectively done in isolation. Even if you are writing a grant for a capstone, thesis, or dissertation (which is expected to be an independent scholarly work), your request for funding is going to involve other individuals beyond you and your supervisory committee. These persons may include study subjects or participants, consultants, institutional review committees, clinical site authorities and personnel, clerical or technical services, and administrative research office personnel. If your grant is not being requested to support your graduate work, it is *expected* that your project will involve a team. How well you choose and assemble a competent, experienced team is the mark of a knowledge-able grant writer and is part of the criteria by which your application will be scored. An interprofessional team is often required for grant submission since the advent in 2009 of the interprofessional education collaborative (IPEC) to encourage interprofessional education and collaborative practice. For more information, see www.ipecollaborative.org/about_ipec.html. The goal of this work and the reason it is tied to research funding is to improve population health outcomes. Funding opportunities for IPEC can be found at www.ipecollaborative .org/funding_opportunities.html with links to the Gordon and Betty Moore Foundation, John A. Harford Foundation, Josiah Macy Jr. Foundation, and Robert Wood Johnson Foundation.

Although not always easy, creating an interprofessional team may broaden populations of interest. Selecting and asking for entrée to conduct your study in a clinical or community study site also involves negotiation with the appropriate personnel. Understanding the importance of these interpersonal links in the grant process not only makes the grant submission process less bumpy, but also ensures a smoother journey throughout the entire preaward and postaward period of your study. Understanding the system by which each group of individuals operates allows you to sufficiently plan your time and procedures.

. . .

YOUR GRANT-CONSTRUCTION TEAM AND SYSTEM

Your grant-construction team can take on a variety of configurations. It may be a capstone, dissertation, or thesis committee; a research team you build from nursing or interprofessional colleagues; or in some instances, a team put together with input from the funding agency.

Capstone, Thesis, or Dissertation Committees

If you are writing a small seed grant, you will likely write the scientific research plan yourself or perhaps write it with the supervision of a capstone, thesis, or dissertation chair; consultant; or statistical advisor. Usually, the largest hurdles in this process are getting the time and help you need from assisting individuals when your grant submission date is growing close. This may have to be orchestrated around receiving institutional review board (IRB) approval from one or more institutions. For example, Kenner had to have her proposal reviewed and approved by her doctoral committee (taking 3 weeks), as well as the associate dean for research where she was on faculty (taking 2 weeks). The IRB for the University Medical Center where she was a student reviewed her proposal, although she was not collecting data there (taking 4 weeks), and finally the hospital IRB where the data were collected had to approve the proposal (taking 4 weeks). The process took 3 to 4 months. She found it helpful to submit each previous letter of approval to the next IRB. Planning ahead, getting firm commitment for appointments, and preparing your agenda and questions prior to each meeting with these members keep your relationships strong and move you ahead. More institutions are attempting to use multi-institutional approvals to fast-track the approval process. This mechanism was created to encourage comparative effectiveness research using large datasets (Paolino et al., 2014).

Larger Grants: More Complex Systems

For larger grants, particularly those with interprofessional partners, your grant writing will be similar to joint authorship. The literary give-and-take must eventually produce a readable plan for meeting the aims and objectives of the grant application. Meeting first to discuss your overall plan gets you all in the same conceptual ballpark. If you, as principal investigator (PI), have specific aims and a short background of the problem, you can ask co-investigators to write parts of the background and significance section for you to include in the grant application. This helps you incorporate additional items in the specific aims section, and your discussion may lead you to add or modify one or more of your aims. At some point, the input of your research site authority, your expert topic consultants, your biostatistician, and your institutional financial office shape the final grant proposal. As PI, your ultimate challenge is to make this plan understandable, cohesive, and acceptable to these individuals, as well as to your funding agency.

Other members of your grant-construction team may include secretarial and financial office assistants. If your grant includes social media, or online components, a person with an instruction technology or instructional design background may be necessary. Remembering that your grant is likely not the only task for which they are responsible, give them your grant submission timeline and allow sufficient lead time for them to respond to your requests. Maintaining excellent relationships with your financial office helps keep communication lines open in the planning and administration of your grant funds. If available, use your institutional accountant to help with budget pages. You must first come up with what you need: personnel and percent effort, equipment type and specifications, types and amounts of supplies, travel, and other technical or episodic services. In large institutions, such as universities, colleges, health science centers, and military installations, your grant must be submitted to an institutional office of research administration (sometimes termed "grants and contracts") to have its budget reviewed and signed off by the institution. Find out before you begin your grant writing what timeline this office requires to sign off on your grant. As institutions across the country have become more research active, the time they require to sign off has lengthened. Some require several days, whereas others require a week or more.

If your project includes human subjects, another part of your grant-construction team is your institution's human research participant protection office or IRB. Developing a continuing relationship with an IRB spokesperson is important for determining the type of IRB review you wish to request and for dealing with future questions that arise during your review. For animal studies, your institution's institutional animal care and use committee (IACUC) serves a similar purpose. In both cases, the IRB and IACUC informs you of any training or preliminary steps that must be taken in using either humans or animals in your study. Know how often these committees meet and what their review cycles are well in advance so that these times can be built into the timeline of grant writing. In the case of nursing research, many healthcare institutions have their own nursing research council that reviews all proposals. This council may be a preliminary step in going to the interdisciplinary IRB, or it may have the authority to be the final approving body. Be sure to find out the steps that are required in your institution for IRB approval.

Last, but certainly not least, keep your dean, director, or supervisor aware of your employment time and institutional resources committed in your proposal. Your employment home is crucial to housing you and your project. Early involvement of your supervisor can avoid snags in the application process or later disappointments if your release time or use of resources is refused. Know the informal and formal politics of who should be notified that a grant is being submitted. For example, most department heads do not like to find out, after the fact, that a grant is being submitted by a departmental faculty member. This is a workforce, not a control, issue. If faculty release time is needed in the grant, supervisors must anticipate the possibility of replacing that person. If a key personnel member is employed outside your institution and has agreed to work on your grant, you should get assurance that they have received internal support for their time commitment. If an "expert" in your institution might feel your grant is in competition with their area or research, consider engaging them in your project or in an advisory capacity. Even having them write a letter of support for the grant would show your respect for their expertise. It is better to find out where you stand on competitive issues before the grant is submitted than to have problems surface when it is funded.

A potential barrier during the summer months, or December holidays, is the unavailability of persons to sign off on grants or to agree to serve on grants. Again, anticipate these scheduling problems early. Check vacation schedules and fit them into the grant timeline. Sometimes, this is not possible if a grant opportunity suddenly arises, but in those rare cases, a designated person usually has signature authority.

* * *

BUILDING A RESEARCH TEAM

Choosing your co-workers for a research study or project is serious business. Aside from choosing people with expertise, you are looking for a cooperative team. A cooperative team will work well under your leadership. There is a line of authority and responsibility in a funded research study that is often overlooked by groups who wish to be democratic and supportive to each member. This resides in the fact that the PI is the person who is ultimately responsible for the conduct of a study, no matter how large or small the size of the team. Even when there are co-investigators on a project, you have administrative authority over the selection of the other team members and the assignment and supervision of their work, as well as responsibility for making sure that the budgeted award is spent correctly and on time. Again, the responsibility rests with the PI to answer scientifically and fiscally to the funding agency.

As PI, you are the leader of the project team. Selecting the key personnel for your grant is like recruiting a winning lineup for a competitive challenge. Each person designated as grant personnel must be justified in terms of the role, preparation for the role, and the amount of time spent in the role. In these times of shrinking grant funds and growing competition, these aspects of the grant proposal are scrutinized closely. Two primary places where role competency and time commitment show up are in the list of key personnel, which includes the percent effort, and in the budget justification. A statement in the budget justification tells reviewers precisely the role that the person will play on the project. A person's preparation for the role appears in the biographical sketches for key personnel, which usually follow those of the PI. If the person has any significant research findings that lay the groundwork for the proposed work, this also demonstrates competency and appears in the preliminary studies section of the proposal.

Be sure to acquaint all members of the research team with what their roles are, how much of a time commitment is involved, and how much, if any, of the grant funds will be used to pay for their time or offset their salaries. This seems like an obvious requirement, but it is surprising how many people forget this information by the time a grant is funded. Some even sign up for other grants and find they are 100% committed elsewhere by the time you are ready to begin your study. Others mistakenly believe they are "funded" on your grant when in fact they have committed their "in kind" participation at no cost. A necessary salary or a large time commitment requires negotiation between the team member and their employer. A sign-off from a department head or agency is one of the documents that your research administration office requires before submitting a grant requiring salary support. If the appropriate people have not signed off for in-kind donation of time and the grant gets forwarded to the office of research administration in the university, college, or hospital, it will more than likely be sent back. If by chance the grant goes to the funding agency without proper sign-off, they also may send it back or just not review the proposal. This is not a time to beg forgiveness later because it can spell disaster for the grant. In some cases, your co-investigator or collaborator may be in a different institution that requires a subcontract. Be sure your key personnel have reviewed and have copies of these documents and review them when your grant is funded.

Key Personnel

Key personnel include the PI, co-investigators, collaborators, research assistants, technicians, data collectors, data managers, and a variety of persons who play an ongoing part on your grant project. In grants that provide salary support, the percent effort and fringe benefits are calculated into the annual budget in detail. Personnel who play an episodic part, such as consultants, transcriptionists, or offsite data analysts, are often paid by the visit or by the hours engaged in the project. As such, they are contracted for the work and paid episodically. It is a function of the pattern of work as much as the type of job that determines this. For example, a graduate research assistant (GRA) may be a key personnel member assigned the work of data entry or data transcription, depending on research training or desire for experience. In some cases, onsite clinical experts may play small but continuing roles as key personnel by serving as consultants. In other cases, these tasks may be allocated to a contracted person by the job.

Co-investigators and Collaborators

Co-investigators and collaborators should represent significant roles on the project, either in intellectual contribution or in oversight of portions of the work. They are often interdisciplinary scientists that offer valuable insight and expertise to the conduct of the study and interpretation of findings. Having interdisciplinary partners is recognized as a strength by the National Institutes of Health (NIH) as they seek applications that facilitate an interdisciplinary research approach that brings together the biological, behavioral, and social sciences to address the nation's most pressing health problems.

Traditional NIH research project grants have a single PI. However, this model does not always work well for multidisciplinary collaborations of various sizes, goals, and disciplines, in which more than one PI would facilitate the project. The title "Co-Principal Investigator" is not used by NIH, but a new NIH model, developed in 2006, would accommodate more than one PI on specific types of grants. These Multiple Principal Investigator awards are designed to support team science and projects with justified expertise (NIH, 2018). However, such grants must justify a compelling rationale for multiple PIs or project directors (PDs), and a leadership plan must be included to show the exact scope of appropriate authority and responsibility, as well as the way that this multiple PI/PD model links to the project aims/goals (NIH, 2016, 2018). The leadership plan includes the governance and organizational structure of the research project, with communication plans and procedures for resolving conflicts. In addition, the administrative, technical, and scientific responsibilities for each specific aim or activity should be delineated for the PIs and other members of the scientific team.

Project Director

PD is a second-level position that is often necessary for a large funded study with salary support. For smaller studies, the role of PD is often taken on by the PI. This is the PI's "right-hand person" in the sense that the role includes supervision of many of the day-to-day tasks. In some cases, the PD recruits and trains the research assistants, sets up meetings for the team, makes rounds to recruit subjects for a clinical study, or is responsible for gathering and managing data collection forms. The variety of tasks involved with a larger project can involve a large amount of effort, so a PD might be hired as a full-time member of the team.

Graduate Research Assistants

GRAs and nonstudent research assistants are important members of your team. They are listed as key personnel if they have an ongoing time commitment for a significant portion of your grant. A GRA can be named in the listing of key personnel. However, if you are not sure who will fill these roles, you may need to put "To be announced" in the space where a name would go. Hiring research assistants after the grant is funded may require checking with your institutional human resource department. Some of the best GRAs for your project may come from students you have mentored or those who apply because they are interested in your research. Although some applicants for research assistant positions may apply because they need part-time work, those who develop an interest in the project are ultimately the best team members. Students can generally be hired with little preliminary advertisement beyond posting a "help wanted" sign. However, nonstudent research assistants usually require placement through your institution's human resource office. Good relationships with research assistants make your project run smoothly. The research assistants deserve good training, good communication channels with the PI, and continued feedback on their performance and contribution.

Consultants

Consultants are a quality check on the scientific conduct of your study. Although previous research and publications help demonstrate the expertise of the research team, consultants can contribute specialized expertise to the project and enhance the overall quality of the proposal. For example, if an infant researcher's expertise is in pain and the proposal is to examine the interface between pain and sleep, adding a consultant with national recognition in infant sleep may strengthen the credibility of the project and enhance its ability to successfully compete for funding. Another example is a study concerning cancer rehabilitation and exercise physiology. For this study, consultants who are expert oncologists coupled with ones who are exercise physiologists are good additions to an academic center grant in which no such expertise is on-site. Statistical consultants may give your team added strength in data analysis and interpretation, as well as help with design sensitivity in your initial planning. Consultants can contribute to the project in a variety of ways, including conceptualization of the study design, selection of research instruments, implementation issues, and data analysis and interpretation. Although consultant costs may vary, provide a detailed description of the consultation services to be rendered, number of days anticipated for consultation, expected rate of compensation, and travel, per diem, and other related costs. Most grants, including NIH applications, require a letter from the consultant confirming their willingness to provide the service. It is important that this letter include the type of service they will provide. Also remember that your agency may require a subcontract and data-use agreement be in place for paid individuals who will serve as consultants or will be involved in data analysis or interpretation.

Specialized Team Members

Specialized team members are persons who can be key personnel if they are serving a continuing role on the project, or if they are working only episodically, they can be listed in the "other" category. These might include data transcriptionists, translators, laboratory technicians, medical device engineers, instrumentation or software trainers, and other experts that are necessary for the conduct of your project.

●　●　●

COMMUNITY-ENGAGEMENT TEAMS

If you are planning a research grant proposal for a project that requires evidence of *community engagement* (i.e., meaningful involvement of patients, caregivers, clinicians, and other healthcare stakeholders throughout the research process), your attention to your research "village" must be even more explicit. Expectations for these grant proposals are to describe how you will involve the community team, from topic selection, through design and conduct of research, to dissemination of results. Greater planning and network development is necessary for community engagement research. More background and details are found in Chapter 6.

. . .

CARE AND FEEDING OF YOUR RESEARCH TEAM

Open communication is the key to caring for your research team. Up-front understanding of each member's responsibilities and chain of communication is crucial. Whereas most of the attention to your team comes after the project is funded, clearly stated expectations should be outlined before a team member is included in your grant application.

Once the grant is funded, you should outline early the expectations for GRAs and other data collectors to attend training sessions and carry out study procedures. Give the entire team telephone, pager, or cell phone numbers to contact a supervisory project person when they are unable to fulfill their work schedule or responsibilities. Transmitting the importance of their contracted participation is essential, particularly for students, who may not realize the seriousness of lost data-collection opportunities that occur when personnel are missing. A communication book is sometimes helpful if there are overlapping shifts of grant personnel working around the clock. In a study of fever in HIV patients, personnel made rounds on each shift to seek participants who had temperature elevations. Each person made notes about potential cases and reported any messages about the study to the next person coming on. The PD checked each day to validate that something was done about requests. Regular meetings, at least monthly, with all personnel keep everyone in touch with the study progress, updates in procedures, and problems that need solving. Mutual respect between every member of the team reinforces a person's value to the study's success. Celebrations and parties help form a collaborative spirit. Taking team members to research conferences makes them feel more a part of the study. We have found that allowing GRAs or other team members to present portions of the study methodology in symposia helped groom them for their own scientific careers. At least three of our GRAs discovered spin-off ideas for their own dissertations from involvement with our study.

Every research team needs training to the specifics of your project. In many cases, this involves training data collectors and PDs to the instrumentation, whether it includes medical devices or test administration. Plan to hold training/demonstrations of how to approach a participant, as well as how to administer a procedure, test, or intervention. Role playing sometimes helps a beginning research assistant. Give constructive feedback with support for areas of weakness and praise for accomplishments.

Make it clear to all participants that the collected data belong to the grant and cannot be used for any other purpose. If delineating the publication plans for your project is not done early in your planning and orientation, you will deal with sticky issues after the fact. Co-investigators can expect to be a co-author in publications arising from a grant project, although this varies across studies. Responsible conduct of research principles calls for authorship to be limited to persons who make a major contribution to concept, design, analysis, and/or interpretation of the work (American Psychological Association, 2016; International Committee of Medical Journal Editors, 2017). This includes participation in drafting the article, revising it critically for important content, and having a voice in its final draft. The PI must decide whether collaborators, experts, research assistants, or consultants are included as co-authors, and their authorship should responsibly be based on their contribution to the project and manuscript. Some journals now require all authors to state their roles and the percentage of work they contributed.

Data collection may require varying amounts of training, and this time should be considered in setting up the timeline of your grant. Recognize that gaining intrarater reliability can take considerable practice and trials before measurement skills are honed and ready for data collection. For example, in a study of drug-induced shivering, we wished to determine if skinfold thickness might be an intervening variable that would influence neural perception of discrepancies between environmental temperature and a rising thermoregulatory set point. An unplanned delay in readying data collection was our lack of awareness of how difficult it was to precisely measure skinfold thickness, even with good instruments. It took approximately 100 trials before our PD gained acceptable intra-rater reliability within her own measurements. In that same study, we found it necessary to train GRAs in proper measurement of tympanic membrane temperatures by first teaching them to use an otoscope to visualize a tympanic membrane. When otoscope visualization was mastered, this in turn rapidly improved their inter-rater reliability in the measurement of tympanic membrane temperatures.

Another area of training that should not be overlooked involves scientific integrity and the importance of maintaining the integrity of the study design. For GRAs and new investigators, impressing on them the importance of finding the *truth*, rather than proving the hypothesis, is essential. Most institutions require that any research personnel be trained by their IRB office and take training in the protection of human research subjects from a recognized service, such as the Collaborative Institutional Training Initiative online program, found at www .citiprogram.org. However, the training in scientific integrity and guarding against fraudulent misconduct in research requires constant reinforcement. Research assistants and colleagues, eager to help their PI succeed, must understand that success is in *finding the truthful answers* to research questions, not in proving that you were right in your hypothetical test.

• • •

DEMONSTRATING LINKS WITH THE COMMUNITY, AGENCY, OR INSTITUTIONAL RESOURCES

Gaining Access

A hallmark of an experienced and competent researcher is the ability to build networks, not only of a strong research team, but also of cooperating community or study site partners. This is not simply a description on paper, but a living breathing network that takes planning, negotiation, and respect for the requested resources. It starts with a request for entrée (power, permission, or liberty to enter). In many situations, starting at the top is essential for gaining authorization to conduct a study in a hospital or clinical agency but recognizing that the persons you may need cooperation from are mid- or service-level providers. It is important to build relationships with these individuals while you wait for formal permissions. Permission to access a military or Veterans Administration facility requires special steps that are formalized with applications, credentialing, and chains of command. Approaching a Native American tribal affiliation also requires meeting with and gaining approval from their governing body, as well as from any local agency or site. Recognizing that you cannot expect rapid access when asking for permission to study a group you are not a part of, successful researchers spend considerable time building relationships with key groups and involving them in participatory roles on the study.

Many successful liaisons are built by having clinical or agency people serve on your study as agency coordinators, inpatient or outpatient clinical site coordinators, or facilitators. Most will agree to serve in this role at no cost, since their duties are limited to making sure your study does not conflict with the daily schedule of the clinical unit or agency. It gives the agency person, often a head nurse or unit manager, close contact with the operations of the study so that they can explain it to other personnel.

Watch Out for Crowds!

As research activity grows in clinical sites, the numbers of studies competing for the same participants grows. Some clinical sites and agencies monitor this and keep the number low to avoid interfering with their operations. Others either do not monitor or are glad for any added interest in their site. One problem with competition for subjects emerged at a public welfare clinic for mothers and infants, which was being used by a nurse researcher with small grant funding. The clinic wrote a support letter for a second researcher employed by the same university as the first, welcoming the project to the site to conduct the study without regard to the study currently taking place. Unfortunately, the second PI also failed to check and discuss the availability of subjects with the first nurse researcher and when a large NIH proposal was funded, it encroached on the existing study. Bad feelings resulted all around and affected relationships between the PIs, the agency, and university research administration. Because no oversight committee at your research site may monitor the use of clients, students, patients, or attendees as research subjects, you should try and find out if other studies are going on and determine if conflicts are likely.

Remembering Where You Are

The research site, whether it is a hospital, clinic, senior center, church, tribal center, or school, is hosting your project and you are the guest. As such, PIs should treat this gift with the respect and consideration it deserves. A spirit of cooperation between others working and studying in the site is far more productive than becoming adversarial over factors that might affect your access. If you anticipate that another study PI is seeking the same type of participants in a different study, try to work this out in a straightforward, but amicable, way. For example, we discovered that a physician was seeking bone marrow transplant patients to study the lymphatic effects of the same drug that caused the drug-induced shivering we were studying. We found it was helpful to include him as an expert on our advisory committee. We also found him willing to cooperate to alternate with us in the acquisition of study participants. In fact, our PD contacted him with participants when it was his turn to accept the next study subject. Whether or not your study is a nursing study, recognizing the interface among medicine, pharmacy, nursing, and agency administration means that you should be respectful and considerate to all who are linked to the patient's care.

Once the grant is funded and procedures begin, the site coordinator can facilitate a time when you can present the study goals to the staff. Keep the staff informed about any changes in your project that would affect your presence, coming and going, from the study site. Be sure that GRAs and on-site grant personnel are introduced to the agency staff. Always be available by phone or pager to the research site in case there are problems with or questions about the study or study participants. Expressions of gratitude to cooperative clinical staff are much appreciated. For example, on national holidays such as Christmas/New Year's Eve, the study team treated each of the clinical research study sites used for the HIV fever study and the drug-induced shivering study with a colorful basket of red delicious apples. Study personnel delivered them to the hospital units and labeled a basket for each shift. Staff also appreciated feeling included in the study by our presentations of study progress and problem solving.

Navigating the Internal Grant Submission System

Each grant writer must determine the internal mechanism for submitting grants, regardless of what type of grant it is. This statement may seem simpleminded, but it is an essential early step in the grant writing process. Many offices and people must sign off on a grant before it is submitted to an IRB or a funding agency. A timeline is needed for staying on target and getting these signoffs early in the writing process.

Some people find creating a flow sheet or a project timeline helpful. Whatever tool is used, determine what steps are necessary before getting too far into the grant writing process. Find out if there are restrictions on how many grants may be submitted in the category in which you are applying. For example, no more than one training grant may be applied for by any institution from the U.S. Department of Health and Human Services in a single funding cycle. Therefore, a clearinghouse in the institution for grant development must make sure that this rule is followed. This clearinghouse may be a center for nursing research, a department-level committee or chair, or the dean's office.

Next, find out who must approve the grant submission and when. Does the project require submission of a concept paper to a department? A training grant may require that the department or curriculum committee see the proposal before any grant is submitted. If approval by the curriculum committee is necessary, find out how often and when they meet, and how long it will take for final approval. Also, carefully read the request for proposals; it may state that a grant must have curriculum, college, or IRB approval prior to submission. For example, the NIH requires that, once the researchers are notified that their grant is within the fundable range, IRB approval must be sought. The NIH regulations further state that no grant award funds are to be released until NIH receives in writing that IRB approval has been obtained.

Early in the grant writing process, determine whether a research office or grants office must oversee or approve the project. If so, this office may have staff and support services that would facilitate the writing process. In addition to providing assistance, the grants office often serves as the final check of the grant before submission. Remember, too, that it is important to know who, outside of the college or institution, must sign off before submission. If the project is a cooperative agreement or if subcontracts must be drawn up for outside personnel to be hired, determine who does this, how long this process takes, and what the procedure is. An external agency that is to supply personnel, as well as the college or grant writer's own institution, often has its own indirect cost rates and financial reviews that produce additional budget pages for your grant. Most will wish to review a grant before submission.

CONCLUSION

The "village" analogy is highly relevant to the grant writing, grant submission, and conduct processes. The diversity of backgrounds, cultures, and competencies is especially heterogeneous in this group. Therefore, communication, respect, and clarity of expectations are key to successful relationships among its members. Choose your team carefully, and take exceptional care of them. They will make you proud! Planning is the name of the game when it comes to internal institutional grant submission procedures and processes. Find out the steps in this process and adhere to them. Always assume that the internal review steps are going to take twice as long as you expect. These steps are important to getting your grant out the door, so don't try to rush them. Finally, remember that your activities aren't the only ones in the village. Avoid traffic jams by planning each step in the submission process before you start your journey.

REFERENCES

American Psychological Association. (2016). Publication practices & responsible authorship. Retrieved from http://www.apa.org/research/responsible/publication

International Committee of Medical Journal Editors. (2017). Defining the role of authors and contributors. Retrieved from http://www.icmje.org/recommendations/browse/roles-and-responsibilities/defining-the-role-of-authors-and-contributors.html

National Institutes of Health. (2016). Write your application. Retrieved from https://grants.nih.gov/grants/how-to-apply-application-guide/format-and-write/write-your-application.htm

National Institutes of Health. (2018). Multiple principal investigators—general information. Retrieved from https://grants.nih.gov/grants/multi_pi/overview.htm

Paolino, A. R., Lauf, S. L., Pieper, L. E., Rowe, J., Vargas, I. M., Goff, M. A., ... Steiner, J. F. (2014). Accelerating regulatory progress in multi-institutional research. eGEMs, 2(1), 1076. doi:10.13063/2327-9214.1076

5

Writing the Research Proposal

WHY THE FUSS ABOUT FORMAT?

It is logical to expect that grant writing guides and workshops have been developed to help with either the conceptual or technical aspects of proposal construction. In truth, both aspects are related and require review and constant update. Some of us become impatient with the ever-changing forms and style changes in grant applications. However, the grant writer should pay some attention to the reasons for the frequency in grant format changes to address them properly in the proposal. Federal grants, particularly those awarded by the National Institutes of Health (NIH), change their formats and areas of emphasis for conceptually valid reasons: to reward *innovation, improve rigor, include diversity, authenticate resources*, and *ensure reproducibility*. As these heightened areas of concern became clear, NIH began to highlight these specific points for investigators. They first began to appear in calls for proposals, and eventually these have been embedded in the format itself, with headings that call for the grant writer to explicitly address each issue. Today's NIH grant reviewers are primed to rate and evaluate the proposal on these specific areas: Significance (including impact and scientific premise), Investigator(s), Innovation, Approach, and Environment. They are also attentive to issues surrounding human subject protections and inclusion of women, children, and minority participants. At the same time, the format of foundation and small seed grants are influenced by the ever-changing formats and emphases mandated for NIH proposals. The key thing to be learned about format is that *change* is the universal constant.

• • •

GRANT FORMAT: SEEKING A FLOW

Beginning grant writers often fall "victim to the dictum" of the required headings in specific grant instructions and formats. Because a grant announcement usually includes a format of headings, the novice tends to believe that it is a type of questionnaire, and all one has to do is fill in the blanks. Failure to recognize section headings as a general road map to guide the logic of a proposal, instead of a checklist, can lead to a choppy collection of information that lacks cohesion and justification. This makes the reviewers' task more difficult in determining what is being proposed, why the project is important, and how the study will achieve its aims. Reviewers are seeking the *flow* between sections and elements of a grant proposal. They can spot an applicant's inexperience immediately when the specific aims page of a grant comes in with nothing else in the section but a list of aims and other sections that seem disconnected from these aims. Explaining the need for logical links is a little like trying to understand physiology from anatomical relationships alone. If you consider the grant *format* as a sequence or order of presentation (anatomical relationships), you see that the format alone does not provide the logical links (interactive relationships) that explain how the sections support and justify one another. Figure 5.1 shows the general anatomy and outline of most grant proposal formats.

Each arrow shows the order each element follows and the items to be included in a particular section, but it does not emphasize the need to show how one link explains the other. Figure 5.2, by contrast, shows how each section explains and justifies each of the following essentials of a successful grant. Not surprisingly, these essentials incorporate the NIH criteria of Significance (including scientific premise and impact), Investigator(s), Innovation, Approach, and Environment:

- Meaningful question (significance, impact, and scientific premise)
- Good science (approach and innovation)
- Careful attention to the application (approach, environment)
- Qualified applicant (investigators)

These elements are not headings in a format, but grant reviewers look for these characteristics as they evaluate your grant.

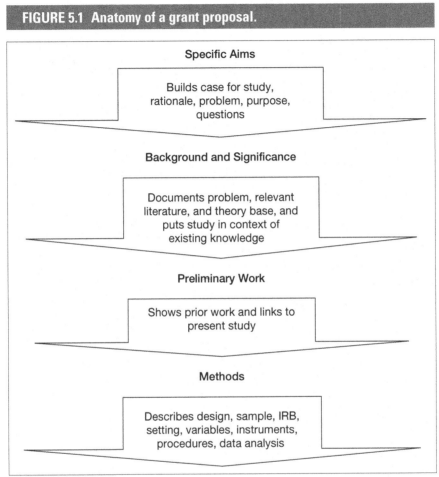

FIGURE 5.1 Anatomy of a grant proposal.

Specific Aims

Builds case for study, rationale, problem, purpose, questions

Background and Significance

Documents problem, relevant literature, and theory base, and puts study in context of existing knowledge

Preliminary Work

Shows prior work and links to present study

Methods

Describes design, sample, IRB, setting, variables, instruments, procedures, data analysis

IRB, institutional review board.

● ● ●

FLESHING OUT THE BLUEPRINT OF A RESEARCH GRANT

The advent of different funding opportunities requiring specific forms makes it more difficult to locate a generic blueprint for today's NIH grants. This makes it essential to find the specific call for proposals or program announcement from the NIH institute website where you intend to apply. Once you have examined the guidelines and format for your intended grant application, you will need to

FIGURE 5.2 Interacting parts of the grant proposal.

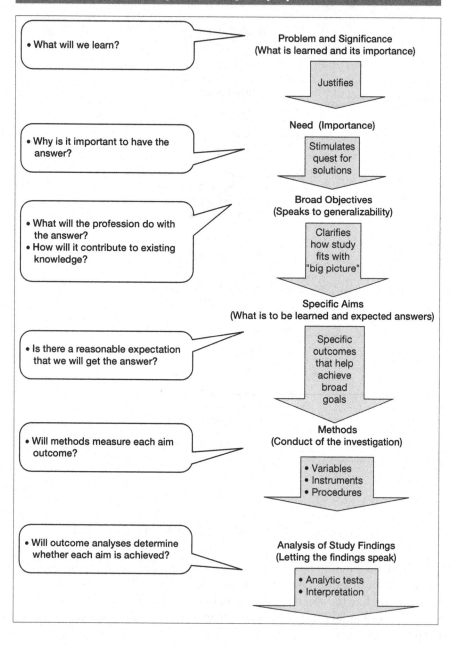

begin constructing your proposal in a well-justified, convincing way. The following is a generic or typical format required by many funding agencies.

Typical Grant Application Format

- Abstract
- Research plan
  - Specific aims
  - Background and significance
  - Preliminary studies
  - Study design and methods
  - Setting and sample
  - Intervention
  - Instruments
  - Data-collection procedures
  - Data analysis
- Time line
- Literature cited
- Budget
- Human subjects considerations: review type and reviewing board
- Appendices

Although nearly all proposals require the information included in this list, the order and specific requirements for *headings* vary by funding agency and sometimes across different funding opportunities within agencies. Clarity and consistency within the grant is one of the major challenges that a grant writer must address. Constructing a research grant application is much like using building blocks: The specific aims form the foundation and structure for the research proposal. From the specific aims emerge testable questions or hypotheses. The study design and methods are then chosen to answer the identified research questions or hypotheses. Appropriate analyses are selected to statistically test hypotheses or systematically answer qualitative questions. One of the ways to promote clarity among hypotheses, variables, instruments, and data analyses is to use consistent vocabulary and terminology among the specific aims, questions/hypotheses, and analytic procedures. Avoid calling a variable by more than one term (e.g., "core temperature" and "central temperature"). Organize each section of the research proposal so that the specific aims are in the same order and sequence as their related questions/hypotheses and plans for analytic procedures. Study variables should also be listed in the same order and sequence in the specific aims, research questions, and hypotheses. The funding agency's application guidelines should include instructions about using special font styles. If the funding agency allows use of special font styles (e.g., bold, underline, or italics), use this feature to highlight key variables throughout each grant section. Finally, well-designed tables and figures can greatly enhance the presentation of materials related to study design and methods.

• • •

COMPONENTS SPECIFIC TO ALL GRANTS

The major components of a research grant application include the following elements that speak to the capability of the investigator(s) and the available resources to carry out the work:

- Abstract
- Research plan
- References
- Budget
- Curriculum vitae, or biographical sketch
- Past and ongoing research support
- Institutional resources
- Institutional review board approvals
- Appendices

The components are not necessarily arranged in this order. Several application formats, including those from the NIH, have the budget and justification pages, biographical sketches, and administrative information in the front. Newer NIH biographical sketches now include research support, which eliminates the older "other support" pages. With newer emphasis on impact, innovation, and rigor, NIH reviewers expect explicit wording highlighting these aspects of the proposal. If your grant allows or requires a section describing institutional resources or available expertise, limit the description to those related to the study.

Although the research grant has been used as the exemplar for this chapter, all elements described here are generally the same with any grant application, including training and special projects. Instead of a research plan, demonstration grants or other project grants may use the terms *plan and implementation*, *project plan*, and *methodology*.

Now that grant applications are being submitted electronically in sections that are already designated, the need for section headings and page numbers on the application are unnecessary. Instead, the submitted pieces are reassembled at NIH and a table of contents and the document is automatically paginated. Newer guidelines for NIH proposals no longer permit information needed to explain a study to be included in the appendix. The lists of typical grant sections and components mentioned earlier in this chapter are general in nature and a good place to start before you know exactly where you will be applying for funds. However, you can no longer assume that the headings and priorities of one agency are the same for another. NIH'S own specifications continue to be driven by priorities. By including the features of the typical grant and highlighting the priorities of the funder, you tailor your proposal to the specific funding opportunity instructions.

Investigate the specific instructions of the particular funding agency you choose before you begin writing. Some instructions limit portions of your grant to specific numbers of pages per section. The title and abstract may be limited to specific numbers of words or characters. NIH has these limitations published in specific website locations (NIH, 2016).

Even if your grant guidelines allow grant proposals to include appendices, do not place information that is critical to understanding your grant there. NIH has become more serious about penalizing attempts by investigators to circumvent page limits by putting essential information for the review into appendices. This improves the grant-review process because reviewers no longer have to flip back and forth between the main body of the proposal and appendices. Therefore, include all the critical information needed to evaluate the quality of the proposal in the Research Plan section of the proposal. Space is at a premium and usually limited to a specific number of pages. The challenge for the grant writer is to present concise, yet detailed plans. Although the format for the research plan may vary depending on the funding source, most research plans include the following sections: Abstract, Specific Aims, Background and Significance, Conceptual Basis of the Research, Preliminary Studies, and Research Plan and Methods: The Approach. The individual sections of a research grant will be discussed in the following subsections.

Abstract

Proposals often begin with a short summary of the proposed research. However, writing the abstract is usually one of the last parts of the proposal you write. A good reason for writing the abstract last is to ensure that any changes that evolve while writing the body of the grant are reflected in the abstract. The abstract briefly introduces the research problem and then summarizes the specific aims, background and significance, and study design and methods sections. The greatest challenge of writing this section is adhering to the word limit. An editor can be extremely useful by helping you cut unnecessary words and phrases. Remember, too, that the abstract sets the stage for the remainder of the proposal. Write with care because the abstract is the introduction to your proposal, and flaws raise questions about your scholarship and set up the proposal for a more critical review. Consistency between the abstract and the remainder of the proposal and your attention to detail help show your capability and "sell" the grant's idea.

Specific Aims

The section called Specific Aims requires a brief introductory explanation describing the study purpose(s), the reasons that it is important to do the study, the potential usefulness of the findings, the intended research accomplishments, and the study's relationship to long-term goals. There is no required order for how the Specific Aims page is written, but proposals in nursing, successfully funded by the National Institute for Nursing Research, tend to follow a favored format. Instead of starting with a list of aims, the elegant Specific Aims page begins with a brief, reasoned argument that (a) poses a problem of relevance to the funding agency, (b) briefly discusses the inadequacy of existing knowledge to address the problem, and (c) sells the need for the proposed research to help fill the knowledge gap. The introductory information helps to "sell" your study idea, and the line of reasoned discussion leads logically into a *statement of the purpose*. The purpose statement should be a concise, clear statement of the study's goal that comes from the study's research problem. It usually includes the relationships sought between the key study variables, as well as the population and setting for the study (Polit & Beck, 2017). In fact, if the introductory discussion is compelling enough, you can begin the statement of the purpose with the words "Therefore, the purpose of the study is…" Here is an example of this approach.

In a funded proposal to study HIV symptom management of HIV-related fever, the introductory paragraph focused on the study problem and factors relevant to fever in HIV infection as follows:

> Fever is one of the most common responses associated with human immunodeficiency virus (HIV) infection, acquired immunodeficiency syndrome (AIDS), and the opportunistic infections accompanying these conditions. Persons living with AIDS (PLWA) experience predictable febrile symptoms, regardless of the infectious agent.[1] Symptoms result from nonspecific and antigen-specific host mechanisms that combat invading microorganisms by activating antibacterial chemical secretion and neutrophil migration.[2] Although T-cell and host immune functions are deranged by HIV infection, proinflammatory responses are activated through alternative complement pathways.[3-4] Whether cytokine-modulated effects related to fever hold immunostimulant benefits for PLWAS is controversial,[5] but the negative effects are well recognized.[1] Pyrogens stimulate hypermetabolic and proteolytic processes that expend oxygen, calories, and body water. In AIDS, these catabolic effects often affect an already compromised nutritional state. Fever is the highest predictor for malnutrition among risk factors in HIV disease.[4] Subjectively, fever symptoms are distressful, interfering with rest, comfort, and functional ability. While medical fever management is understandably concerned with control of the underlying infection with drugs, nursing fever management is directed at symptomatology, regardless of etiology. Goals are to maintain body temperature within a safe

range, maintain and restore fluid balance, conserve energy, avoid fatigue, and promote thermal comfort during fever.

Following the introductory statement, the study problem is discussed in light of existing knowledge as follows:

Although nurses devote hundreds of hours daily to treatment and palliation of fever, care methods have changed little over the past century. Nurses tend to monitor fever progress following pharmaceutical prescriptions strictly, while resorting to poorly justified nursing activities to cool the patient without regard for expected physiologic responses. Effects of environmental temperature, patient hydration, and physical activity on febrile responses are seldom considered. Only recently have specific interventions for fever management been tested, and these have yet to find their way into nursing textbooks.[6-8] Aggressive efforts to cool febrile patients by convective heat-exchange and ice packs are counterproductive because they stimulate shivering and vasoconstriction. Compensatory warming responses generate and conserve heat, increasing oxygen consumption 3–5 fold.[9] Anemic, weak, and cachectic patients tolerate exertion of febrile shivering poorly, as respiratory rate, heart rate, and blood pressure rise to meet oxygen demands.[8] Fatigue, dyspnea, and aching muscles follow shaking chills in febrile immunosuppressed cancer patients.[10]

The next part of the paragraph emphasizes the *need* for the study and the proposed solution:

Interventions are needed that (a) promote heat loss, without inducing compensatory warming mechanisms, (b) promote energy conservation and restoration through rest and control of shivering, and (c) restabilize hypothalamic thermostatic control functions through rehydration and antipyretic drug therapy. Therefore, this study will test effectiveness of a structured protocol to modify thermoregulatory responses during various phases (chill, plateau, or defervescence) of the febrile episode by use of (a) nonpharmacological, scientifically based interventions to control chills and febrile shivering at the onset of temperature spikes and during warranted cooling procedures, (b) warmth, insulation, and convection control to reduce reactivation of chills during the "warm" phases of the febrile episode, and (c) a regimen of nonsteroidal antipyretic therapy and fluid restoration during the febrile episode.

Finally, the intent of the proposal becomes highly focused and specific as it ends with the aims. Each aim is elaborated with the appropriate hypothesis or research question relating to it. The accepted abbreviation for hypothesis H is used with a subscript of its number. Sometimes a research question is more appropriate than a hypothesis, so in that case an acceptable abbreviation of R is used instead with a subscript of its number:

Specific aims are to test the efficacy of a structured protocol during acute febrile episodes in PLWAS to:

1. Reduce frequency, severity, duration, and reactivation of shivering during fever episodes.
   H_1 Febrile shivering episodes are less frequent, severe, and of shorter duration with extremity wraps than without.
2. Reduce distress, chill perception, and fatigue associated with the chill phase of fever.
   H_2 Visual Analog Scales for distress, chill, and fatigue perceptions during chill phase of fever are less with extremity wraps than without.
3. Influence cardiorespiratory indicators of exertion during febrile episodes.
   H_3 Elevations of BP, RPP, and respiratory rate during febrile episodes are less with extremity wraps than without.
4. Influence body temperature patterns and variability during febrile episodes.
   H_4 Body temperature elevations are less severe and shorter with extremity wraps than without.
5. Control shivering when aggressive cooling treatments are warranted.
   H_5 Shivering activity is less frequent or severe during surface cooling with use of extremity wraps than without.
6. Maintain body hydration during febrile episodes.
   H_6 Skin and mucous membrane hydration and daily body weight are more stable with a fluid protocol than without.

By leading into the purpose statement with your persuasive introduction, your reviewers will find it easier to see the logical link between the need and the solution (your proposal). This also means that the last thing they will read before leaving the page is the list of specific aims, their related hypotheses, and questions. All of the cited examples must appear on one page in NIH grant applications, which can be seen in Exhibit 5.1.

In summary, the goals of the NIH research proposal should be of major significance in terms of the health of the people of the United States. Well-developed specific aims should logically follow and flow from your study goals and purpose and be clear, concise, attainable, and distinct from one another. A well-written Specific Aims section is crucial and should guide the study design and methods.

Background and Significance

Traditionally, the Background and Significance section of a grant connects a proposed study to what is known about the problem. It familiarizes the reviewer with the documented research findings about the problem and discusses your

EXHIBIT 5.1 Example of an NIH Specific Aims Page

Specific Aims: Fever is one of the most common responses associated with human immunodeficiency virus (HIV) infection, acquired immunodeficiency syndrome (AIDS), and the opportunistic infections accompanying these conditions. Persons living with AIDS (PLWA) experience predictable febrile symptoms, regardless of the infectious agent.[1] Symptoms result from nonspecific and antigen-specific host mechanisms that combat invading microorganisms by activating antibacterial chemical secretion and neutrophil migration.[2] Although T-cell and host immune functions are deranged by HIV infection, proinflammatory responses are activated through alternative complement pathways.[3-4] Whether cytokine-modulated effects related to fever hold immunostimulant benefits for PLWAS is controversial,[5] but the negative effects are well recognized.[1] Pyrogens stimulate hypermetabolic and proteolytic processes that expend oxygen, calories, and body water. In AIDS, these catabolic effects often affect an already compromised nutritional state. Fever is the highest predictor for malnutrition among risk factors in HIV disease.[4] Subjectively, fever symptoms are distressful, interfering with rest, comfort, and functional ability. While medical fever management is understandably concerned with control of the underlying infection with drugs, nursing fever management is directed at symptomatology, regardless of etiology. Goals are to maintain body temperature within a safe range, maintain and restore fluid balance, conserve energy, avoid fatigue, and promote thermal comfort during fever. Although nurses devote hundreds of hours daily to treatment and palliation of fever, care methods have changed little over the past century. Nurses tend to monitor fever progress following pharmaceutical prescriptions strictly, while resorting to poorly justified nursing activities to cool the patient without regard for expected physiologic responses. Effects of environmental temperature, patient hydration, and physical activity on febrile responses are seldom considered. Only recently have specific interventions for fever management been tested, and these have yet to find their way into nursing textbooks.[6-8] Aggressive efforts to cool febrile patients by convective heat-exchange and ice packs are counterproductive because they stimulate shivering and vasoconstriction. Compensatory warming responses generate and conserve heat, increasing oxygen consumption 3–5 fold.[9] Anemic, weak, and cachectic patients tolerate exertion of febrile shivering poorly, as respiratory rate, heart rate, and blood pressure rise to meet oxygen demands.[8] Fatigue, dyspnea, and aching muscles follow shaking chills in febrile immunosuppressed cancer patients.[10] Interventions are needed that 1) promote heat loss, without inducing compensatory warming mechanisms, 2) promote energy conservation and restoration through rest and control of shivering, and 3) restabilize hypothalamic thermostatic control functions through rehydration and antipyretic drug therapy. Therefore, this study will test effectiveness of a structured protocol to modify thermoregulatory responses during various phases (chill, plateau, or defervescence) of the febrile episode by use of 1) nonpharmacological, scientifically based interventions to control chills and febrile shivering at the onset of temperature spikes and during warranted cooling procedures, 2) warmth, insulation and convection control to reduce reactivation of chills

(continued)

EXHIBIT 5.1 Example of an NIH Specific Aims Page (*continued*)

during the "warm" phases of the febrile episode, and 3) a regimen of nonsteroidal antipyretic therapy and fluid restoration during the febrile episode.

Specific aims are to test the efficacy of a structured protocol during acute febrile episodes in PLWAS to:

1. Reduce frequency, severity, duration, and reactivation of shivering during fever episodes.
   H_1 Febrile shivering episodes are less frequent, severe, and of shorter duration with extremity
   wraps than without.
2. Reduce distress, chill perception and fatigue associated with the chill phase of fever.
   H_2 VAS distress, chill, and fatigue perceptions during chill phase of fever are less with extremity
   wraps than without.
3. Influence cardiorespiratory indicators of exertion during febrile episodes.
   H_3 Elevations of BP, RPP, and respiratory rate during febrile episodes are less with extremity wraps than without.
4. Influence body temperature patterns and variability during febrile episodes.
   H_4 Body temperature elevations are less severe and shorter with extremity wraps than without.
5. Control shivering when aggressive cooling treatments are warranted.
   H_5 Shivering activity is less frequent or severe during surface cooling with use of extremity wraps than without.
6. Maintain body hydration during febrile episodes.
   H_6 Skin and mucous membrane hydration and daily body weight are more stable with fluid protocol than without.

Source: Holtzclaw, B. J. (1994). Febrile symptom management for persons living with AIDS (R01 NR03988). Bethesda, MD: National Institute of Health, National Institute for Nursing Research.

study in light of the existing knowledge. However, interpretations of significance in grant applications need to fit closely with a funding agency's mission. In 2010, NIH announced the intent to enhance review criteria for research applications and require investigators to be clearer about the expected outcomes of their research. The criteria for significance became more specific to whether the project addressed an important problem or a critical barrier to progress in the field. In addition, the assessed overall *impact* of a study would become a recognized scoring element. *Impact* was defined as the assessment of the likelihood for the project to exert a sustained, powerful influence on the research field(s) involved. This is another area where logical flow is extremely important because the significance of your research is determined by how it confirms, refutes, or fills a gap in what is currently known. It is important to convince the readers that this study is the next logical step based on the state of the science. It is also important to show how this research addresses a widespread or significant health concern. Linking your proposed research to national health objectives such as *Healthy People 2020* and *2030* (www.healthypeople.gov) or a professional organization's research priorities strengthen the likelihood of funding for the proposed research.

The Background and Significance section in NIH grants is where *relevant literature* and the conceptual or theoretical framework of the study are reviewed. Even if another grant application format calls for a section titled "Literature Review," this section should be written carefully and succinctly to display the strengths or weaknesses of the existing knowledge. The review should be balanced, revealing evidence that both supports and disputes your proposed hypotheses. Be assured that at least one of your grant reviewers will be familiar enough with the literature to find any existing evidence you might have overlooked. A well-written Background and Significance section displays your familiarity with the area and its underlying scientific base. Review of relevant literature about the study's phenomenon of interest (e.g., pain) informs the reviewer of how existing knowledge supports the study design, methods, or approach.

Although today's grant applications tend to limit extensive literature reviews, the growing emphasis on evidence-based practice has stimulated a proliferation of integrative reviews on specific topics. These reviews can provide in-depth resources for grant writers seeking to justify a proposed area of study, intervention, or educational program. Systematic or integrated reviews are available on the Internet in databases such as the Cochrane Collaborative, Vermont Oxford Network, or specific topic reviews or implementation reports such as the Joanna Briggs Institute. These databases are repositories for findings and reviews of different levels of research but primarily contain randomized clinical control trials. The information available from these integrated reviews provides a strong foundation for your study's question, research plan, and background and significance sections of your grant application. You may find that your own search and integrative review of literature provides you a better tailor-made explanation of your study phenomenon. In either case, the literature reviewed to support your proposal should be both relevant and current. Move beyond simply summarizing the literature in your proposal to critically evaluating existing knowledge and identifying gaps in the scientific evidence. After all, if the existing literature is complete and has no gaps or controversies, you will have a more difficult time justifying why your study is needed. Likewise, if you present only the literature that supports your view, your reviewers may decide you are either biased or uninformed.

Conceptual Basis of the Research

Today's NIH grants are expected to be justified by a *scientific premise* that is defended by sound rationale. The scientific premise helps support the significance of the project and should be clearly identified in your proposal. The logic of your scientific premise, supported by its study's scientific or conceptual underpinnings, helps reviewers see how it could influence the concepts, methods, technologies, treatments, services, or preventative interventions that advance your field. Even theory-generating, qualitative, or naturalistic research is *informed* by the investigator's ideas or by the context in which it is studied to determine what, and under what conditions, it is to be studied. In quantitative research, the conceptual links between variables, even the variables themselves, originate in the context of existing knowledge. If the study is quantitative with descriptive or manipulated variables, the idea for why you should be collecting them is driven by observed or theoretical connections. Conceptual frameworks may be highly formalized and "named," or they may be constructed logically from commonly accepted principles of psychology, physiology, physics, or other sciences. In any case, the conceptual basis for your proposed research should be stated clearly and identified and accompany the review of relevant literature. Once you have identified a conceptual model or theoretical basis for your questions, these concepts must be connected to your research plan. Grant reviewers look for how the framework of your study drives or explains the relationships you are studying. Explain and clarify how the relevant concepts are empirically evidenced in your study. If a conceptual framework is used, it should not only be clearly tied to the present study, but also be well mapped to other parts of the application. A diagram of a conceptual framework is a visual way of demonstrating relationships that are known and relationships that have not been investigated and may be the focus of your study. Finally, the Background and Significance section should clearly support the specific aims of the study. As with the specific aims, this section is a reasoned argument, justifying the need and importance of your study. For example, if your study's conceptual framework is based on the Whole Person Suffering Model, each of the four areas (physical, psychological, spiritual, and social) should be addressed in the review of relevant literature.

Preliminary Studies

Depending on the specific format of your selected funding agency, you may not always have a specific section that allows you to showcase explicit evidence of your qualifications in the proposal itself. This is true of NIH grant applications that, because of space limitations, have incorporated some aspects of preliminary studies into the revised biographical sketch and others into the significance section. Preliminary data can be used to build a case that your earlier research and preliminary findings have led you to the current investigation. This work can support feasibility of your specific aims and testability of hypotheses. Novel findings from your preliminary work can also strengthen the Approach section of your Research Plan and be used in justifying the methodology. Be sure to include any relevant information that highlights your qualifications to carry out the proposed study in your biographical sketch. Tailor your biographical sketch to highlight relevant accomplishments. These may not always be the same depending on the funding agency. Remember too that the grant proposal is a marketing piece to showcase how good you are and how you are the perfect person or team to carry out the work. This is not the time to be modest.

Research Plan and Methods: The Approach

The research plan is the "meat" of a research proposal, and the *design and methods* section includes the methodological portion of the proposal. As such, it is the most critical component of the proposal. The research plan should be clear, concise, and cogent and contain sufficient information for the reviewers to evaluate the proposal.

The NIH has identified the research proposal's plan and overall strategy, methodology, and analyses as the *approach*. Approach is a criterion assessed by grant reviewers to ensure that your proposal uses a strong and unbiased approach that justifies feasibility, weighs alternative approaches, and manages protection against risk.

In NIH grants, the Research Plan includes the following:

- Study Design
- Setting and Sample (including inclusion/exclusion criteria and sample size justification)
- Intervention Protocols or Experimental Conditions (if relevant)
- Variables, Measurements, and Instruments
- Data-Collection Procedures
- Data Analyses
- Study Time Line

Study Design

The study design is the "blueprint" or strategic plan that the researcher uses to accomplish the specific aims and answer or test the research questions and hypotheses. Research proposals should explicitly describe the design to be used. Depending on how complicated your plans are, your description may entail using a different approach for each of your specific aims.

There are several ways to categorize study design. In the past, most research methodology was categorized as either quantitative or qualitative. However, these terms are very nonspecific and primarily refer to the type of data rather than the actual study design. Some experts assert that the more accurate terms are *naturalistic* and *positivistic* designs in which qualitative or quantitative data are collected (Tripp-Reimer & Kelley, 2006). As new design strategies developed to meet unique research needs, textbooks and researchers began to use the terms *quantitative* and *qualitative* as *approaches* rather than designs.

In each global category (naturalistic, positivistic, qualitative, quantitative), there are more specific terms that fine-tune the approach and more completely inform the grant reviewer of the type of design you plan to use. In some situations, you may wish to examine a cross-section of the population, correlating one variable with another to test one specific aim. In the same study you may wish to collect repeated measures of a variable over time to test another specific aim. Sometimes a researcher may wish to examine a phenomenon both quantitatively and qualitatively to meet the needs of a particular research study.

Quantitative Data

Quantitative data are analyzed using statistical methodology that focuses on counting or quantifying data by defining, measuring, and analyzing them. The research questions answered by this method are concerned with describing quantifiable attributes, finding relationships, causality between variables, and predicting outcomes. Statistics are used to summarize data, determine sampling error that could influence the findings, and test hypotheses. The study design using quantitative data can be further classified by the terms *descriptive* or *observational*, *case*, *time sequenced* or *longitudinal*, *prospective*, *retrospective*, *experimental*, and *quasiexperimental*. The gold standard for experimental studies remains the randomized controlled trial, but most clinical studies use quasiexperimental designs because the clinical situation makes it difficult to meet the three criteria for experimental research: (a) manipulation, (b) randomization, and (c) control. Quasiexperimental research may often lack a control group, random selection, random assignment, or active manipulation. The fact that research subjects are free to refuse or withdraw from participation in a study limits randomization considerably.

Qualitative Data

Qualitative data collected by naturalistic approaches are used to describe the nature or meaning of "what is" according to the person or phenomenon being studied. Although many descriptions and definitions exist describing qualitative research, six characteristics defined by Speziale and Carpenter (2007, p. 21) illustrate important features of researchers who use qualitative approaches: (a) a belief in multiple realities, (b) a commitment to identifying an approach to understanding that supports the phenomenon studied, (c) a commitment to the participant's point of view, (d) the conduct of inquiry in a way that limits disruption of the natural context of the phenomena of interest, (e) acknowledged participation of the researcher in the research process, and (f) the reporting of the data in a literary style rich with participant commentaries.

The most often used approaches to collecting qualitative data include ethnography, grounded theory, and phenomenology. However, case study methods, hermeneutics, oral histories, and critical, philosophical, and historical approaches to inquiry are emerging, along with their own set of undergirding philosophies, theoretical perspectives, and approaches for collecting and analyzing data (Tripp-Reimer & Kelley, 2006). Naturalistic research seeks an in-depth understanding of a phenomenon that pays particular attention to its contextual nature. The *inductive* characteristics of this type of research often yield rich data that inform science about the meaning of a situation. Newer approaches have combined both qualitative and quantitative forms in *mixed methods*. Mixed methods is not a patchwork mixing of study findings, but rather involves the philosophical assumptions and use of both qualitative and quantitative approaches, and integration of them, in the study. Mixed methods purpose statements and research questions must clearly identify sufficient information about the quantitative and qualitative elements of the study to provide rationale for using both to answer the research objectives (Creswell, 2014). A comparison of qualitative, quantitative, and mixed methods from Creswell's textbook on this topic appears in Table 5.1.

TABLE 5.1

QUANTITATIVE, MIXED, AND QUALITATIVE METHODS

Quantitative Methods	Mixed Methods	Qualitative Methods
Predetermined	Both predetermined and emerging	Emerging
Instrument-based questions	Both open- and closed-ended questions	Open-ended questions
Performance data, attitude data, observational data, and census data	Multiple forms of data drawing on all possibilities	Interview data, observation data, document data, and audiovisual data
Statistical analysis	Statistical and text analysis	Text and image analysis
Statistical interpretation	Across databases interpretation	Themes, patterns interpretation

Source: Creswell, J. W. (2014). *Research design: Qualitative, quantitative, and mixed methods approaches* (4th ed., p. 17). Thousand Oaks, CA: Sage.

It is beyond the scope of this book to provide detailed descriptions of design methodologies. Each design has a different goal, and the best design for your study is the one that flows logically from the problem statement, literature review, theoretical framework, and research question or hypothesis. The choice of a study design is a major research decision because each requires familiarity and skills with its unique data-collection, data-management, and analytic approaches. Keeping these ideas in mind, you should use the strongest study design feasible to maximize the credibility and dependability of the study findings. In addition, the selection of credible and capable consultants to help you navigate your chosen study design and statistical analyses strengthens the research grant proposal.

Examples of both qualitative and quantitative research data were used in Kenner et al.'s study (1990) "Transition from Hospital to Home for Mothers and Babies from Levels I, II, & III Nurseries." She first wanted to find out, "What was it like for a mother taking a baby home from a neonatal unit?" "What concerns or problems did the mothers have during the first and fourth weeks at home with the baby?" and finally "What could we have done differently at the hospital to ease the transition to home?" She used a phenomenological approach to gather these data, gathering qualitative data in three different settings. From these data, she developed a transition questionnaire on the basis of the five categories of concern that evolved from the qualitative studies. The transition questionnaire was a quantifiable tool used to measure the phenomenon of transition. Although she was still concerned with the three original research questions, Kenner then used the transition questionnaire to quantify the mothers' responses.

Once the study design is chosen, the researcher should clearly describe the design and methods as well as the rationale for selection. In many studies, a quasiexperimental design is chosen over a stronger true experimental design because of the inability to physically or ethically manipulate certain variables. These variables include elements such as overall environmental lighting, the heating level within an incubator, and responses to prescribed medications.

The researcher should articulate other designs that were considered and the rationale for why the proposed study design is superior to alternative designs. For example, instead of a clinical trial with an experimental and a control group, a repeated measures design where patients serve as their own control may be justified by the ability to control for possible contamination by variability between participants. In the use of a crossover design, this same justification is used, but with the added benefit of controlling for *order effects* by having half the subjects exposed to an intervention and half in the control group, then switching the groups to the opposite condition (treatment/control). If a third trial is used, the groups are switched back to the original condition. In a study of the efficacy of wrapping extremities to prevent drug-induced febrile shivering, Holtzclaw used a crossover model (Figure 5.3). Although the strength of this model was the control

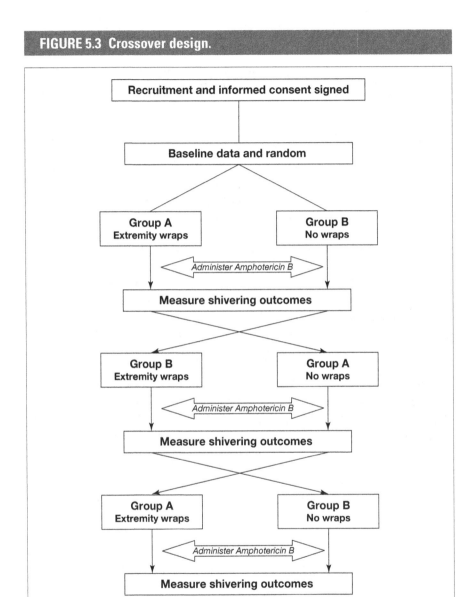

FIGURE 5.3 Crossover design.

for subject variability between treatment and control conditions and the control for order effects, the design was not without limitations. This design required a 10-day "washout" period to remove any carryover effects of the intervention and involved the participation of each participant in the study for a longer time. Each of these limitations were anticipated and justified in the proposal.

Clearly state the assumptions and limitations of the proposed research. If problems are anticipated, possible solutions or strategies should be discussed to minimize their occurrence. For example, in longitudinal studies, subject attrition is expected, and the principal investigator (PI) should include a discussion of strategies to maintain subject participation over time.

Setting and Sample

Provide a description of the setting chosen for the study along with the rationale for its selection. Describe in detail the type of setting, location, and typical patient population. Selection of this setting over other possible ones must be specifically stated and convincing. Furthermore, if you select a distant site instead of a local site, it is important that you provide a rationale for that decision. Address how distance will affect data collection and quality of data-collection methods. For instance, the grant writer may describe a plan for the selection of a site coordinator employed by the clinical agency or one who lives close to the site as a strategy to handle the issue of distance. The proposal must also address plans for ensuring appropriate training and reliability of research assistants, and it must address plans to monitor the site to ensure the integrity of data-collection methods. Finally, the researcher must document that the research site is willing to provide the researcher with access to subjects. This is usually best accomplished by submitting letters of support from key personnel at the study site, such as the medical director, nursing director, or other applicable administrative personnel. If you have chosen a study site in a hospital, clinic, educational institution, or organizational setting, you should anticipate the need to show entrée, access, or permission to use that site. In many grant proposals, including NIH applications, reviewers look for letters of agreement or approval to conduct the study in these sites.

Clearly describe the criteria for inclusion and exclusion of subjects in the study. Depending on the space available in the grant application, the grant writer must describe more fully why these criteria were selected and how they help control for threats to external validity. In addition, the researcher has an obligation to convince the reviewer of the adequacy of the site to produce a sufficient number of subjects on the basis of inclusion and exclusion criteria. To address this issue, include in narrative text or table format the number of subjects who meet the inclusion criteria and who are available per month or year for study at the data-collection site. In addition to the number of subjects, federal grants now require that the PI address the recruitment of special populations, including gender and racial/ethnic groups, as well as women and children. Federal grants also require a completed Targeted/Planned Enrollment Table (see the section on inclusion of women, children, and minorities).

The sample size of the proposed study is also important to emphasize. As discussed in Chapter 2, a power analysis should be performed to justify the proposed sample size. The power estimate justifies the sample size needed to avoid drawing a conclusion with findings that occurred by chance alone. For a grant proposal, reviewers want to know the factors you have considered in arriving at that number. That is, you must make clear the *level of significance*, the *desired power*, and the *expected effect size* used in the power analysis. Because the calculated *p* value of your findings reflects the probability that a significant finding occurred by chance *alone*, the level of significance (*p* value) is usually set at less than .05 (the lower the *p* value, the lower the likelihood of the finding happening by chance). The power estimate and significance criterion are set a priori (before beginning the study). Base the sample size on the most conservative number needed to answer the research question or hypothesis being proposed. For example, if you plan to use both hierarchical regression and repeated measures analysis of variance (ANOVA) statistics in your study, base your sample size on the number needed to achieve the desired power for *each* analysis. The researcher should also discuss how sample size is adjusted to account for subject attrition. For example, in a previous pilot study, if 15% attrition was noted due to mortality of subjects, the sampling plan is adjusted to oversample by 15%.

Sample selection strategies and group-assignment protocols should be explained. Two groups of sampling techniques used in nursing research are probability (random) sampling and nonprobability (nonrandom) sampling. Random sampling techniques are preferred and result in more representative samples; nonprobability sampling techniques are more feasible, practical, and economical. Variations on *simple random sampling* include *stratified random sampling*, *cluster sampling*, and *systematic sampling*. All of these strategies depend on having access to all members of a given population from which the sample will be drawn. Although random sampling is difficult to achieve in clinical settings, *random assignment* to groups is often easily accomplished. Subjects can be randomly assigned to treatment conditions by using methods such as flipping a coin, pulling slips from a hat, or, more commonly, a table of random numbers.

Nonprobability sampling is frequently used in beginning studies because individuals are found in the situation or location that is accessible. The *convenience sample*, also called *accidental* or *incidental sample*, is an example in which participants are included because they happen to be there and because there is generally less cost involved in finding them. The biases possible with such sampling should be recognized and any anticipated influence on study outcomes acknowledged. For example, possible biases influencing an intervention study may be linked to the likelihood of greater motivation among people who volunteer for studies.

Intervention Protocols or Experimental Conditions

If an intervention or experimental study is proposed, the grant proposal should clearly describe the intervention protocol and the rationale supporting the expected outcome. Describe how the intervention is administered in detail. Include how the treatment condition differs from the control or comparison group. For major grants, pilot testing of the intervention is expected before the grant. All NIH grants expect some preliminary work to support an intervention, even for a pilot study. However, some foundations and granting agencies accept proposals for early pilot work if sufficient evidence from the literature or observations shows a strong possibility that an intervention might be effective. Once the pilot is completed, the data form the foundation for larger, more competitive grants. If your research proposal does not involve an intervention protocol, this section is omitted.

An example of an intervention protocol is found in Holtzclaw's HIV symptom management study testing the efficacy of extremity wraps to prevent febrile shivering (Holtzclaw, 1994):

> *Intervention Protocol*: The treatment condition for this study involves the use of warmth, insulation, and protection from sensed heat loss throughout the febrile period, while allowing heat excesses to be lost from areas that do not trigger warming responses. Abrupt temperature elevations indicate fever "spike" (> 1°C within 1 hour). The control group is monitored without extremity wraps. Wraps are applied to the treatment group according to the following protocol:
>
> 1. Apply monitoring electrodes, blood pressure cuff, and temperature probes prior to wrapping procedures.
> 2. Place three bath towels lengthwise under each arm. Bring up lateral edges of towels to form a seam. Secure with plastic clips along seam. Allow intravenous lines, monitor leads, and blood pressure tubing to exit along seam. Roll up excess toweling at fingertips to form a "mitten." Secure with tape.
> 3. Place three bath towels lengthwise under each leg. Bring up lateral edges of towels to form a seam. Secure with plastic clips along seam. Allowing monitor leads to exit along seam. Roll up excess toweling at toes to form a "boot." Secure with tape.
> 4. Take care to avoid overlapping excess toweling against extremity in order to maintain consistency of insulation.
> 5. Do not allow towels to remain damp. If sweating is excessive or towels become damp, replace quickly with warmed towels causing as little exposure or air movement as possible. Note time and length of exposure on the record.

Variables, Measurements, and Instruments

The researcher should provide operational definitions for each of the independent and dependent variables within the proposed study. Study variables can also be clarified in a table format that matches each of the independent and dependent variables to a particular instrument or subscale on an instrument. For pen-and-pencil questionnaires, describe the population, method of administration, reliability, and validity for each instrument used. For scientific devices, provide information as to the accuracy, precision, range, and reliability. Specialized devices and laboratory assays may have specific qualities, such as collection condition, temperature, and linearity requirements. *Variables* are logically associated with the *instruments* used to measure them in a research study. If space is at a premium in your grant application, it may be to your advantage to deal with them together by stating the variable, its measurement modality, and the company or author of the instrument. However, if specifications of the instruments are complex, you may need to operationalize each variable, ascribing its measurement modality, but follow with a detailed separate section called "Instruments."

The following example uses separate variable and instrument sections:

Variables: The following independent variables are under study: The *independent variable* in each case is the study protocol implemented at the fever onset. Contained in the protocol are (1) *documented fever spike* measured by a >1°C rise in temperature within 1 hour; (2) *insulative extremity wraps* to protect dominant heat loss skin sensors in arms, legs, hands, and feet (see Tables 1 and 2); (3) *warm liquids* given in metered amounts, in insulated cups; and (4) *acetaminophen* 650 mg given every 4 hours for temperature >39°C. The *dependent variables* to be measured are (1) *shivering* measured for <u>onset</u> by prototypic phasic masseter electromyographic (EMG) signals, (2) *severity* by an ordinal scale 0–4 and actigraph signal on the multichannel monitor indicating extremity involvement, and (3) *duration* by timing from onset to end with a sweep second-hand stopwatch. *Chill perception* and *thermal distress* will be measured on two separate visual analog scales measuring these related but different subjective responses to sensed changes in temperature. *Fatigue* will also be measured by visual analog scale. *Heart rate* will be monitored by the multichannel monitor, as will *skin temperatures* and *aural canal* temperatures. *Blood pressure* will be measured by battery-powered automatic self-inflating blood pressure cuff and recorded by the observer. *Respiratory rate* will also be a variable observed by the data collector. *Core temperature* will be measured from the tympanic membrane by a handheld infrared light reflectance thermometer by the data collector. *Water loss* will be measured by 24-hour *weight loss*, by *observed sweating severity* on an ordinal scale, and by *dehydration severity* on an ordinal scale.

Instruments and Data Collection Procedures: Shivering stages will be measured on an ordinal *severity scale* of 0–4, with each stage representing extension of shivering to progressively larger muscle groups. Based on work by Hemingway, which demonstrated shivering follows a cephalad-to-caudal progression, with earliest hard-to-detect tremors beginning in the masseters, and most violent shivering including the extremities, a scale has been refined by Abbey[26] and adapted for nursing studies.[8,31,41] In the inpatient setting, stages will be verified by the following:

> 0 = No shivering activity. Absence of phasic bursts on EMG and no palpable or visible muscle fasciculation found by nurse observer.
>
> 1 = Masseter contractions measured by EMG and nursing observations. Light touch over mandibular angle reveals vibration to fingertips of examiner. This hard-to-detect tremor precedes shivering and any significant effects on oxygen consumption.[35]
>
> 2 = Face and neck contractions observed by investigator.[26,41] In clinical studies, this stage was accompanied by significant increases in metabolic rate and oxygen consumption.[35]
>
> 3 = Pectoral contractions extend to abdomen, palpation of abdomen reveals involvement of lower trunk, extremity movement is *passive* (assessed by grasping elbow and wrist).
>
> 4 = Generalized shivering, measured by nursing observations of generalized rigor and bed shaking contractions, teeth chattering. Signaled by Actigraph on the multichannel monitor. Described as the highest muscle involvement in shivering. Extremities *actively* contract.

Electromyogram: Nursing observations and EMG monitoring will be continuous. Onset and stage 1 will be verified by masseter EMG activity. Although implanted needle electrodes are more sensitive, they are rejected for use with immunosuppressed patients because they penetrate skin and subject patients to infection and bleeding. Disadvantages of surface electrodes include lack of discrimination between muscles and lack of sensitivity in measuring activity levels in deep or small muscles. Interference from electrical environment is also problematic. Surface measurements are satisfactory, however, when general information about onset and severity of shivering is required, particularly when the patient is under bedclothes. For maximum sensitivity, electrodes will be placed as close as possible to the middle of the muscle belly. Shivering activity has been noted to differ from artifact or purposive movement in its pattern and amplitude of EMG recordings. Short phasic bursts in the 100–500 microvolt range characterize masseter contractions during shivering.[35,41] A portable electromyogram designed specifically for facial muscle contractions (Myotronics, Inc., Seattle, WA) will be used at the bedside. Data are collected via a Dolch portable microcomputer at the bedside. The software package captures EMG tracings over time, averages signals every 15 seconds, and graphs every 30 seconds. The event marker allows recording of other phenomenon occurring at any given point in time. Involvement of extremities in shivering will also be assessed by means of the *movement actigraph*, a motion-sensitive wristband device attached to the Mini Logger II multichannel monitor.

Temperature measurement: Core temperature will be measured by infrared light reflectance tympanic membrane thermometer (Genius; Intelligent Medical

Systems, Carlsbad, CA). This nonintrusive measurement is safe, rapid, and found accurate within .1°C and accurate up to 40.5°C in vitro in our preliminary work. During training for previous studies, in vivo interrater and intrarater reliability was within .1°C after training to use the device with ear tug and "otoscope" approach. Use of continuous temperature monitoring with the Mini Logger II will record three sites of skin temperature (for calculation of *mean skin temperature*) and *aural canal temperature*, on separate channels for storage in computerized memory that can be downloaded to the investigator's microcomputer. Disposable temperature probes (YSI 400, Yellow Springs, OH) with self-adhering contacts will be applied to the lateral thigh, approximately half the distance between knee and hip joints. *Heart rate* (HR) will also be obtained by cardiac monitor from another channel on the Mini Logger II. Self-adhering silver/silver chloride electrodes will be applied to the chest and a flexible chest band applied to maintain contact. HR will be used with *blood pressure*, obtained from the automatic, battery-powered, oscillometric blood pressure cuff (Dynamap, Critikon, Tampa, FL) to calculate *rate pressure product* (RPP). RPP provides an indirect estimate of myocardial oxygen consumption and cardiac effort.[42] The *Mini Logger II* multichannel unit combines temperature, activity, and HR monitoring capability into a single compact unit. The unit is a refinement of the Mini Logger I, adding HR and an event marker. The basic unit has been a reliable, accurate, and rugged instrument for use in the field. The temperature units can be verified by water bath calibration to confirm accuracy (Appendix H). *Body water loss* will be measured by three criteria: (1) physical assessment of skin moisture and turgor, (2) eyeball depression by gentle touch, and (3) dry tongue used to rate dehydration on an ordinal scale of 1 to 10, with 10 being extremely desiccated and 0 being well hydrated. *Sweating severity* will be rated on a 0–4 ordinal scale, with 0 = dry to touch, 1 = moist to touch, 2 = beads of sweat on brow and upper lip, 3 = sweat running down face and neck and spotting clothing, and 4 = clothes saturated with sweat. *Body weight* will be measured every day at the same time on a clinical balance scale. *Visual Analog Scales* (VAS): (Appendix H) will be administered by the investigator and include *thermal perception* (TP-VAS), meaning whether a person feels warm or cold, and *thermal comfort* (TC-VAS), meaning how comfortable a person is at that temperature. Subjects are asked to mark on a 100-mm line, bounded on each end by a descriptor. For thermal perception, the descriptors are "as cold as possible" and "as hot as possible," respectively. For thermal comfort, the descriptors are "intense discomfort" on one end and "extreme comfort" on the other. The scale is scored by measuring the distance in millimeters from 0 at the cold end to the patient's mark, somewhere between 0 and 100 mm. VAS have been used in assessing a variety of subjective states.[43] This scale was found to have construct validity and criterion validity with extant measures of thermal comfort used by environmental engineers.[44] *Fatigue* will be measured by the VAS for Fatigue (VAS-F) developed by Lee, Hicks, and Nino-Murcia.

It is a VAS with 18 items that includes fatigue and energy subscales. It was found to be a valid and reliable VAS for normal and patient populations.[45]

Justifying Alternate Instruments: If alternate instruments are available or more traditionally used, the applicant will need to discuss the rationale for the selection of a particular instrument. A sample rationale for studying pain from an R15 application follows (Walden, 2001):

> Pain research has produced several valid and reliable pain instruments, including the CRIES (Krechel & Bildner, 1995) and the Premature Infant Pain Profile (PIPP; Stevens et al., 1996). While the CRIES has been validated for use in infants greater than 32 weeks gestational age, the PIPP can be used in preterm infants below 28 weeks gestational age. Furthermore, the PIPP is preferred over the CRIES in this study as it controls for two significant contextual factors (gestational age and behavioral state) known to modify pain expression in preterm neonates (Craig et al. 1993; Grunau & Craig 1987; Johnston et al. 1993; Stevens & Johnston 1994; Stevens, Johnston, & Horton 1994; Stevens et al. 1993; Johnston et al. 1999). The PIPP will be used to measure acute pain response in this study.

Describe any necessary training of research personnel in the use of each instrument. The researcher should report pilot data or if any is planned for new instruments. Finally, include copies of all instruments in an appendix.

Data-Collection Procedures

The description of study procedures usually begins with a clear description of how potential subjects are identified and recruited as participants into the study. This is often followed by a clear description of how and when the intervention will be carried out. Provide the method of data collection and how often measurements are recorded. Include aspects of how, when, where, and who uses the instruments. If other study personnel are involved in data collection, a description of their training should be included. Describe the methods used to ensure inter-rater reliability. The researcher should address any problems that may be encountered during the study protocol and include the plan for how the problems will be addressed. If the study is complex, a step-by-step procedural checklist should be developed and used by data collectors to ensure that no procedural item is omitted during the course of the study. If a checklist is used to simplify data-collection procedures, include this checklist as an appendix for the reviewers to examine.

Finally, use diagrams of the data-collection procedure to clarify the study design and timing of data collection for study instruments. For example, the following diagram (Figure 5.4) was used to illustrate the data-collection procedures for the variables contained in the pain study (Walden, 2001).

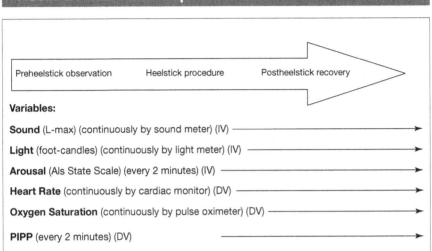

FIGURE 5.4 Data-collection protocol.

Sample: Gestational age groups: 25–27 weeks (n = 51), 34–36 weeks (*n* = 51).
DV, dependent variable; IV, independent variable; PIPP, Premature Infant Pain Profile

Data Analyses

The data-analysis section should provide a clear description of plans for data management, refinement, and reduction. Proposals often adequately address the plans for statistical analyses but fail to provide sufficient detail on how large, complex data sets will be reduced for analyses. The researcher should therefore take great care in describing how data will be collated, coded, keyed, and verified.

Base the selection of the statistical analyses on the level and type of data. Furthermore, the statistical analyses should match the specific aims and research questions or hypotheses. Organizing the presentation of data in this section by specific research question or hypothesis is often helpful for both the grant writer and reviewer. Constructing a table that shows each aim and its related hypothesis, the variables and instruments to measure them, the level of measurement for each variable, and the statistical test for each hypothesis is an excellent way of organizing this presentation. The PI would be wise to include a biostatistician on the research team. Involve the biostatistician early to assist with the development of the statistical plan of the study, including design, analyses, and plan for dissemination of project findings. Often, a biostatistician has the best knowledge and expertise to write the data-analysis section of a proposal that involves biological assays, unusual statistics (such as those used in circadian rhythm measurements or genetics), or covariates of various variables (see the Sample Research Plan for examples of data analyses).

Study Time Line

The time line is used to provide an anticipated time frame for project activities, including start-up activities such as hiring and training of project personnel, identification of subjects, data collection, data preparation and analysis, and report writing. Be realistic in your time frame; projects always take longer than you expect. It is better to project a longer time for a certain aspect of the grant, say the hiring of personnel, so that you will have some extra time when other aspects of the grant take longer than expected. This information can be provided in narrative form, or the grant writer may choose to present this section in the form of time line table. Time lines can be simple with broad categories of activities listed (see Figure 5.5), or they can show phases and changes in personnel mandated by a more complicated study.

References

The references, or Literature Cited section, is the final part of your research plan and contains references to journal articles, books, and other materials that *you have cited* in your grant proposal. Check for any inaccuracies and correct them. Reviewers may retrieve literature you cite to verify your interpretation. Be sure to check the URL links on any references you have retrieved from the Internet. These sometimes change or become inactive between the time you accessed them and the time you prepare your proposal. Complete bibliographical information should be provided using a consistent referencing format, such as the American Psychological Association. If you have used a superscript-style reference format such as that required by the *Journal of the American Medical Association*, your reference list will be numbered in the exact order the references appeared in your proposal. This method saves you much-needed space in the proposal and is a favorite among NIH grant applicants. If you use a superscript-style reference format, make sure you verify your references before you submit your final grant because their numbering may have changed during grant editing.

Budget

The first important task in creating a budget for the proposal is to review the funding agency's budget criteria closely. The funding agency usually specifies

FIGURE 5.5 Timeline for a 3-year grant.

Grant Year	Year 01												Year 02												Year 03											
Grant Month	1	2	3	4	5	6	7	8	9	10	11	12	1	2	3	4	5	6	7	8	9	10	11	12	1	2	3	4	5	6	7	8	9	10	11	12
Calendar Year	2018												2019												2020											2021
Calendar Month	4	5	6	7	8	9	10	11	12	1	2	3	4	5	6	7	8	9	10	11	12	1	2	3	4	5	6	7	8	9	10	11	12	1	2	3
Ordering Supplies	▓	▓																																		
Hiring Personnel			▓																																	
Training Personnel				▓																																
Subject Recruitment						▓	▓	▓	▓	▓	▓	▓	▓	▓	▓	▓																				
Data Collection								▓	▓	▓	▓	▓	▓	▓	▓	▓	▓	▓	▓	▓	▓	▓	▓	▓	▓	▓										
Data Analysis																									▓	▓	▓	▓	▓							
Research Consultant									▓						▓					▓				▓					▓							
Data Interpretation																														▓	▓	▓	▓			
Writing Reports																																	▓	▓	▓	▓

what expenses are allowable and what is not fundable. For example, some grants do not allow for the salary of the PI, but do allow salaries allocated for consultants and research assistants. Some federal grants do not allow for travel costs related to dissemination, whereas others may. Foundation grants typically do not pay as high a rate of facilities and administrative (F&A) costs as federal grants. In fact, some pay none at all. If you are in an academic institution, part of your preparation for applying for a foundation grant is to clarify F&A questions and possibly negotiate a waiver of the established institutional rate. If this is not possible, you will need to pay these administrative costs out of your grant budget. It is therefore extremely important to have a clear idea about the funding guidelines before you start to develop your budget for the proposal.

If you are in an academic center, there may be research offices with personnel specifically trained to assist you in preparing the budget. The highly experienced staff in these offices can help you obtain salary information, benefit costs, cost of common budget items such as equipment, computers, pagers, mileage, and other costs. Salaries often are the largest budget item. For each person listed on the grant, indicate the percentage of commitment to the grant and their salary and fringe benefits. The budget office will assist you in computing indirect costs and setting up subcontracts with other institutions.

Clearly match budget items to grant activities (research personnel, consultants, equipment, supplies, travel, computer costs, and other related expenses). The goal is to ask for what you need to conduct the study. Most funding agencies require a budget justification for grant expenses. Budget justification is a specific description of each of the budget items requested and a rationale for why this expense is needed. Appropriate budget planning will help you budget appropriately while avoiding the tendency to pad the budget. Although money can often shift within the same category of the budget, often the budget does not allow shifting of monies between categories, such as salary dollars and equipment costs. Therefore, carefully consider where the monies are allocated within the budget.

Federal agencies often use a modular budget process for grant applications requesting up to $250,000 in direct costs per year. For these applications, total direct costs for the proposed study typically are divided into modules of $25,000. Although a standard modular grant application requests the same number of modules in each year of the grant, additional narrative budget justification is required if researchers wish to request variation in the number of modules requested. For example, if the grant involves the purchase of expensive physiological data-acquisition equipment, the PI may want to provide additional budget narrative to explain an increased number of modules for the first year of the grant. Investigators should review other specific features of the modular research grant, particularly if changes in activity or personnel are anticipated in the final years (NIH, 2017).

The "cost of doing business" in carrying out a project of any kind often gets too little attention. As a result, there is sometimes a mismatch between what you need and what you've requested. It is never a good idea to skimp on the budget with the notion that it makes the grant more fundable. The contrary is true. Grant reviewers will likely see that you have no idea of how much support it takes to carry out the proposed work. On the other hand, reviewers are on guard for attempts to pad a budget. Salaries are likely to be the highest expenditure on extramural grant budgets, and PIs often cuts corners on their own salary so that colleagues can be included as co-investigators or travel to meetings can be included to present their work. This is foolhardy and can jeopardize your review. If you are funded with such poor planning, you will find that your work is not compensated for in your budget. Map out the chores to be done on the grant, and figure as closely as possible how much time it will take you and your team to carry out the work. Request salary support for this amount and provide the rationale for each.

Budgeting salaries for smaller federal proposals, such as R03 and R15 grants, takes careful consideration. Salaries can take up much of a modular budget with a maximum allowable budget cap. Therefore, it is prudent to not allocate personnel positions when they are not needed. For example, if you are collecting samples that can be frozen for a laboratory assay, you could hire a laboratory technician near the end of the study. If you are using research assistants to collect data, you would not need their services during the last few months of the study, when reports and analytic interpretation take place. These time-limited salaried positions can be shown clearly on your grant time line and the rationale included in the budget justification.

Another misconception of novice researchers is that the indirect costs associated with the grant are taken out of the regular grant budget. The reality in most situations is that these are funds "in addition" to the grant budget and are designed to cover operating or overhead costs. The amount or percentage of indirect costs is determined by the funding agency and the researcher's institution. Some funding agencies do not pay indirect costs, and this must be negotiated with the employing institution. Not all institutions encourage researchers to apply for funds when no indirect costs are possible. For example, indirect cost "exception forms" for grants at the University of Oklahoma College of Nursing must be approved by the college dean and then forwarded for signature of the vice president for research at the health sciences campus.

Finally, remember to update the budget as revisions are made throughout the grant writing process to ensure the consistency of the proposal to funding requested. For example, if the sample size changes and thus the amount of time needed to pay a research assistant changes, adjust the budget to reflect these changes.

Human Subjects Considerations/Human Welfare Protection

This grant section should provide a clear description of procedures for protecting subjects' rights and obtaining informed consent. Discuss measures to protect anonymity or confidentiality related to data collection, management, and storage. Identify potential risks and anticipated benefits of the study. Fully describe potential risks, measures to minimize those risks, and institutional resources available to treat clients who develop health-related complications that arise as a result of the study. Indicate whether the institutional review board (IRB) approval process is complete or pending.

Institutional Review Board Approvals

An IRB is a panel of health professionals across disciplines and at least one or two consumers. This panel is charged with reviewing any protocol that will be part of a research study involving humans. The IRB must ensure scientific merit and protection of human subjects. The IRB must question whether a study is ethical regarding the protection of human subjects. As shocking as this is to us today, in the 1940s, prisoners were used in studies to determine how infectious diseases progressed. These studies were later deemed unethical because a captive population was used. Prisoners were probably coerced into participating, and they were not informed of potential life-threatening dangers. Today an IRB would prevent this study from taking place. The IRB exists strictly to protect a person's rights and safety in any research study. IRB approval is an expectation for any grant award, and in most institutions, studies are not allowed, even as staff projects, without IRB approval. The IRB reviews informed consent forms. The forms must be written at a low reading level (ideally third grade, but no higher than fifth or sixth grade), understandable to the population being tested, and in most instances, translated into the population's native language. Protection of human subjects and disclosure of the intervention are important aspects of this process.

Timing of IRB Approvals

Today, IRB approval is not required before NIH peer review of an application. Because fewer than half of all applications submitted to NIH are funded, the policy was modified to reduce the burden on applicants and submitting institutions. However, no grant award can be made without IRB approval. Applicants and research institutional offices have online access to their peer-review scores and approval progress through the NIH Electronic Research Administration Commons (eRA Commons). Therefore, following NIH peer-review and notification-of-priority score/percentile, institutions should proceed with IRB review for those applications that have not yet received IRB approval and that appear to be in a fundable range.

If the research is a multisite/institution study, more IRBs are accepting an approval from one institution to another. In other words, if the PI receives IRB approval at one institution, the next institution may accept this as its own approval. For example, comparative effectiveness research generally requires multiple sites to answer the research question. To ensure timely approvals in such cases, collaboration, including regulatory approvals, is needed (Paolino et al., 2014). The researcher needs to check with the local IRB to see what rules apply for multisite studies. Institutions may also require data use agreements be in place to share data between institutions in multisite studies. The researcher should check with his or her legal or research-compliance office to determine what agreements are required.

NIH Policies Affecting Human Subjects

Some of the most significant changes affecting NIH grant applications have been in the area of human subjects. Legislation and policies that protect and allow more inclusiveness have created new section headings, review criteria, and oversight. It is therefore prudent to review these policies and grant application forms at the NIH website (www.nih.gov) to determine whether you have the latest information. Your office of research administration will also be helpful in directing you to recently emerging new policies. The following subsections discuss several changes that are already in effect.

Data Safety and Monitoring Plan

In 1998, the NIH issued a policy stating that any research involving a clinical trial or intervention must have provision for data and safety monitoring to protect participants from physical and psychological injury or violations of privacy. Monitoring should be commensurate with the size and complexity of the project. This means that a smaller project could be monitored by individuals or a committee, and a large multisite project would engage a national committee. The complexity of a large phase III clinical trial requires independent data and safety monitoring. If your study does not entail a clinical trial or test of an intervention, state so in this section of your grant application. However, it is also prudent to add that you are monitoring the progress of the study for adverse events and have a plan of action to address such possibilities. Describe the mechanism for reporting adverse events to the IRB, FDA, and NIH program official responsible for the grant. Finally, include in your proposal your plans for ensuring data accuracy and study protocol compliance.

Inclusion of Women, Children, and Minorities

During the past two decades, it has become clear to the scientific community that most clinical research findings have been based on studies of adult white men. As more evidence emerged about genetic and gender-based differences in response to therapy, it became clear that treatment responses based on research done on one population subgroup might lead to poor treatment choices in other groups. Today, several groups—women, children, and minorities—are actively included in all NIH-funded studies unless their exclusion is scientifically justified. The cost of including these groups is not considered an adequate reason for exclusion. If inclusion is expected to be difficult, a plan for recruitment is required.

In 1993, the NIH Revitalization Act wrote into law measures ensuring that women and members of minority groups are included as subjects in each project of clinical research. Amendments to this legislation were made in 2001 to clarify when and for what purpose modifications can be made. It remains the policy of NIH that women and members of minority groups and their subpopulations must be included in all NIH-funded clinical research, unless a clear and compelling rationale and justification establishes to the satisfaction of the relevant NIH institute/center director that such inclusion is inappropriate with respect to the health of the subjects or the purpose of the research. Exceptions are frequently requested to study a disorder (e.g., prostate disease or ovarian cancer) that is specific to one gender or to study problems that are specific to a subpopulation.

An NIH policy on the inclusion of children in clinical research was developed in 1998 because medical treatments applied to children were too often based on adult testing. The tendency to exclude children from research studies meant that their treatment was not scientifically evaluated for their age or development level. The policy states that children (persons under the age of 21) must be included in all human subjects' research conducted or supported by the NIH, unless there are scientific and ethical reasons not to include them.

Targeted/Planned Enrollment Table

To facilitate your completing the section on inclusion of women and minorities, a "Targeted/Planned Enrollment Table" is required in a section of your NIH grant dealing with recruitment. Your planned enrollment should be based on some scientific approach, whether it is to try to duplicate the proportions of each minority category in a region or to ensure an equal number in a comparative study. There must first be a *plan* to include the targeted individuals (recruitment strategies, inclusion of additional sites if necessary, targeting under-represented agencies). Your table should reflect that plan. All your planned participants are first divided into ethnic categories by gender. Ethnic categories in the table are (a) Hispanic or Latino, and (b) not Hispanic or Latino. Participants are then divided into racial categories by gender. Racial categories are (a) American

Indian/Alaska Native, (b) Asian, (c) Native Hawaiian or other Pacific Islander, (d) Black or African American, and (e) White. Done correctly, you will have the same totals in each category division.

Animal Welfare Protection

Applications that involve research with animals go through a different ethical review process by an organization's institutional animal care and use committee (IACUC). This committee is as rigorous and concerned about animal welfare as the IRB is about the welfare of humans. Animal use protocols generally require a lay explanation of the project, animal methods to be used, a description of surgical procedures that will be performed, a justification of animal numbers, a list of any hazardous and controlled substances, and a section on considerations of alternatives to animal use for the purposes of minimization of animal pain and distress. Before being approved by the IACUC to conduct research involving animals, the PI and study team is typically required to complete animal-certification training, a health screening, and relevant Collaborative Institutional Training Initiative online modules.

Newer guidelines from the NIH ask applicants to check "Yes" to the question, "Is the IACUC review pending?" even if the IACUC review/approval process has not yet begun at the time of submission. Even though an IACUC approval date is not required at the time of submission, this and other data may be requested later in the pre-award cycle. Because getting IACUC approval requires steps of training and review, it is prudent to submit the review request in a timely manner to avoid any delay in the grant-review and award process. Just as the IRB approval must precede any research funding concerning humans, no grant award for animal research can take place unless IACUC approval is made.

Appendices

Appendices supplement key information contained within the research plan. Not all funding agencies accept appendices. In addition, not all reviewers at the discussion table receive them. NIH rulings limit investigators from circumventing rigid space limitations in proposals by adding essential information in appendices, so do not give in to this inclination. Ensure that both the abstract and the research plan include *all* pertinent information by which the scientific quality of the proposed study is to be evaluated. When they are allowed, the appropriate use of appendices may greatly enhance the research proposal submitted for review by allowing the applicant to provide examples of scholarly writings that show previous relevant work. Nearly all funding agencies allow and expect inclusion of data-collection or biomedical instruments to be used in the research. Schematics for an elaborate study apparatus or a biomedical device that might interrupt the flow of the study description are often placed in the appendix. However, simple line drawings and conceptual maps that clarify your study belong in the body of the research plan. Other items commonly included in the appendices are letters of support from consultants and clinical agencies and subject consent forms.

CONCLUSION

There are several aspects that characterize a good grant proposal. First, a good grant proposal is based on a creative, well-articulated research question and on a significant health issue. For an educational or a special-projects grant, the proposal must articulate the need and the potential pool of students or persons served. Second, the grant must be methodologically sound, well written, and carefully formatted. The presentation should convince reviewers that the research team is highly knowledgeable about the topic and possesses the necessary skills in research methods to expertly carry out the proposed work. Finally, the grant writer must check and recheck the proposal to ensure consistency from specific aims, research questions and hypotheses, background and significance, study design and methods, data analyses, and proposed budget. The same checklist holds true for educational grants, but the terminology changes to goals and program objectives for the specific aims and research questions. The study design becomes program design, and the data analysis must have a strong program-evaluation component with clearly articulated outcome metrics. The budget would be the same type as for research projects. Do not assume that the reviewers will know what you mean. Putting on the hat of the reviewer versus that of the writer may help clarify issues throughout the proposal that require further explanation.

> *"Do not write so that you can be understood; write so that you cannot be misunderstood."*
>
> —*Epictetus*

REFERENCES

Creswell, J. W. (2014). *Research design: Qualitative, quantitative, and mixed methods approaches* (4th ed.). Thousand Oaks CA: Sage.

Holtzclaw, B. J. (1994). Febrile symptom management for persons living with AIDS (R01 NR03988). Bethesda, MD: National Institute of Health, National Institute for Nursing Research.

Kenner, C., Flandermeyer, A., Hadley, B. J., Kotagal, U., Thornburg, P. D., Berns, S. P., & Spiering, K. (1990). Transition from hospital to home for mothers and babies from levels I, II, & III nurseries. Grant funded by University of Cincinnati College of Nursing & Health Research Challenge. National Association of Neonatal Nurses.

National Institutes of Health. (2010). Enhancing peer review: The NIH announces enhanced review criteria for evaluation of research applications received for potential FY2010 funding. Notice Number: NOT-OD-09-025, Bethesda, MD: Author. Retrieved from https://grants.nih.gov/grants/guide/notice-files/not-od-09-025.html

National Institutes of Health. (2016). Page limits. *Grants and Funding*. Retrieved from https://grants.nih.gov/grants/how-to-apply-application-guide/format-and-write/page-limits.htm#other

National Institutes of Health. (2017). NIH modular research grant applications. *Grants and Funding*. Retrieved from https://grants.nih.gov/grants/how-to-apply-application-guide/format-and-write/develop-your-budget/modular.htm

Paolino, A. R., Lauf, S. L., Pieper, L. E., Rowe, J., Vargas, I. M., Goff, M. A., ... Steiner, J. F. (2014). Accelerating regulatory progress in multi-institutional research. eGEMs, 2(1), 1076. Retrieved from https://www.ncbi.nlm.nih.gov/pmc/articles/PMC4371517/

Polit, D. F., & Beck, C. T. (2017). *Nursing research: Generating and assessing evidence for nursing practice* (10th ed.). Philadelphia, PA: Lippincott Williams & Wilkins.

Speziale, H. J. S., & Carpenter, D. R. (2007). *Qualitative research in nursing: Advancing the humanistic imperative* (4th ed.). Philadelphia, PA: Wolters Kluwer/Lippincott Williams & Wilkins.

Tripp-Reimer, T., & Kelley, L. S. (2006). Qualitative research. In J. Fitzpatrick & M. Wallace (Eds.), *Encyclopedia of nursing research* (2nd ed., pp. 497–499). New York, NY: Springer Publishing.

Walden, M. (2001). Environment and sleep on preterm infants' pain response. Bethesda, MD: National Health Institute, National Institute for Nursing Research (R15 NR007731-01).

6

· · ·

Engaging Communities in Research Grant Development

· · ·

GET READY FOR A DIFFERENT APPROACH!

This chapter presents grant writing guidance in the context of community-engaged research or collaborative community partnerships. This topic is timely and particularly relevant to emerging funding opportunities. Among the federal initiatives committed to community engagement (CE) are the Clinical and Translational Science Awards (CTSA), the NIH-funded Research Centers in Minority Institutions Program, the prevention research centers in the Centers for Disease Control and Prevention (CDC), and the Agency for Healthcare Research and Quality (AHRQ) practice-based networks. Grant application requirements have moved beyond community-informed or community-based involvement to *community engagement* with documented commitment of all involved in the partnership and specific mandates for shared decision making and resources. Recent announcements by health experts and health system research funders document the importance of CE grant writing competence in ensuring competitive proposals (National Academies of Sciences, Engineering, and Medicine, 2017; Sheridan, Schrandt, Forsythe, Hilliard, & Paez, 2017; Talib et al., 2017). In addition to federal funding agencies, foundation funders, such as Susan G. Komen, mark as a priority the authenticated engagement of community-based stakeholders in awarding their breast cancer project grants.

• • •

CAN YOUR PILOT STUDY BUILD CAPACITY FOR CE?

If you are just beginning pilot work or a preliminary study that depends on group participation, you may recognize that you are also beginning to build a community alliance or network. Positive relationships with community partners in small projects can be steps toward laying the foundation for strong long-term projects in the future. Working with collaborative partners gives you and your partner valuable experience in cooperative planning strategies that will be useful for future, more formalized networks. Just as "partners" were emphasized as evidence of a competent investigator in Chapter 2, your pilot funding and joint scholarship becomes permanent evidence of your enduring collaborative relationships for subsequent grant proposals (Holtzclaw, 2007). Community partners are equally important as indicators of existing and ongoing relationships in community-engaged research. As you plan for and promote partnerships for future funding opportunities, take the opportunity to partner with volunteers, community representatives, and other collaborators from your pilot work in your presentations and publications. Joint authorship and public recognition acknowledges the importance of these individuals and helps you document existing collaborations as you seek further CE funding mechanisms.

When partnering with community members who are new to the research and project development, you as a leader must empower them early by building their capacity to participate. This calls for providing training and resources, as well as a clear definition of roles for all participants.

• • •

ORIGINS OF COMMUNITY-BASED EFFORTS

Community involvement in improving health is not a new idea. In fact, it has been an accepted cornerstone of public health for many years. The success of these efforts is seen more recently in the engagement and joint efforts of communities, families, and interested stakeholders with academic and scientific researchers to address key health concerns for cancer prevention, smoking cessation, obesity, and heart disease. Although community-based participatory research (CBPR) efforts have improved environmental and resource-management problems for some time, the benefits of an equitable partnership approach became more widely recognized by healthcare as principles of CBPR were developed (Horowitz, Robinson, & Seifer, 2009; Israel et al., 2008; Israel, Schulz, Parker, & Becker, 2001). However, this general familiarity with community involvement has not necessarily informed the public and organized medicine about the differences between "community-based" and "community-engaged," where engagement can be viewed as a continuum from consultative to cooperative to collaborative, based on involvement in a commitment to a partnership or program (CTSA, 2011). Although attractive in its philosophy and relevance to the needs of the community, the implementation of full CE requires careful planning and a full understanding by participants of what the commitment to a partnership approach means. Partnership research equitably involves community members, organizational representatives, and researchers in all aspects of the research process in which all partners contribute expertise and share decision making and ownership. This approach is not necessarily intuitive, and it is not feasible without some general principles, organization, and acknowledgment that all participants have something of value to contribute. These factors should imply a long-term relationship, not a quick match aimed at making a project attractive to a recent call for proposals. Rather, such projects should emerge from an existing relationship between an educational or clinical entity and a community of interested stakeholders (e.g., public health agencies, practice-based researchers in clinics, organizations, nursing homes, policy makers, parents, family, community associations). Partnerships drawn from these organizations are more likely to succeed if grounded in principles of community organization: "fairness, justice, empowerment, participation, and self-determination" (CTSA, 2011). A wealth of informative resources is available at minimal or no cost through NIH publications and reports. A recommended primer as you start this work is *Key Principles of Community Engagement*, 2nd ed., produced by the CTSA Consortium (Department of Health and Human Services, NIH, CDC; Agency for Toxic Substances and Disease Registry, and CTSA; CTSA, 2011). There have been sufficient teams trained by funding agencies to provide useful, experience-based tips in carrying out CE research, so workshops and orientation events are well worth the time to attend. Encouraging as many diverse members of your own team to become oriented also has lasting effects.

* * *

WRITING A GRANT PROPOSAL FOR CE: A DIFFERENT APPROACH

CE research has traditionally been patient or population centered, but a growing emphasis of this approach is on having communities play a part in answering "real questions in real time" to improve decision making (Institute of Medicine, 2011, p. 165). Traditionally, research approaches warranted having systems gather data in large centralized databases to be analyzed over years by scientists who are remote from the healthcare situation. A different approach is seen in CE in which a network of information and analytical tools is developed, enabling clinicians and community participants to analyze research evidence in the context of their own locality and in real time. Although many basic principles and elements of grant writing apply to forms and applications for CE proposals, "different approach" factors include the community-relevance assumptions underlying research questions, their significance to stakeholders, and the practicality it offers them.

* * *

WHAT IS YOUR COMMUNITY?

Funding agencies want clear descriptions of the group with which the project is engaged (Patient-Centered Outcomes Research Institute [PCORI], 2016). Is it a localized community, including all of those living within its boundaries, or is it a community that is defined in some other way? Old definitions of community requiring a formal or geographical identity may no longer apply to the community you wish to work with. This is because community can be described from at least four perspectives: (a) a systems or organizational perspective; (b) a social perspective composed of social and political networks; (c) a virtual perspective enabled by modern technology through computer-mediated communication that no longer keeps persons place bound; and (d) an individual perspective that relates to a person's identity or sense of membership that also enables individuals to belong to more than one community at a time (CTSA, 2011). A community can be any group of people who work collaboratively with a common interest or goal. This diversity in perceptions of community was predicted by the CDC'S 1997 definition of *community engagement* as "The process of working collaboratively with and through groups of people affiliated by geographic proximity, special interest or similar situations to address issues affecting the well-being of those people" (CDC, 1997, p. 9).

* * *

WHAT LEVEL OF CE ARE YOU SEEKING FOR YOUR PROPOSAL?

As funding mechanisms and agencies have become more specific in their requirements for proposals to state the explicit community you wish to engage, they also expect to know what level of engagement you propose. Your proposal must therefore be more competitive if you identify potential challenges that accompany each increasing level of community involvement. Figure 6.1 shows each level of involvement along with the increasing potential for challenges at each level (CTSA, 2011).

FIGURE 6.1 Community engagement continuum

Outreach	Consult	Involve	Collaborate	Shared leadership
Some community involvement.	More community involvement.	Better community involvement.	Community involvement.	Strong bidirectional relationship.
Communication flows from one to the other, to inform.	Communication flows to the community and then back, answer seeking.	Communication flows both ways, participatory form of communication.	Communication flow is bidirectional.	Final decision making is at community level.
Provides community with information.	Gets information or feed-back from the community.	Involves more participation with community on issues.	Forms partnerships with community on each aspect of project from development to solution.	Entities have formed strong partnership structures.
Entities coexist.	Entities share information.	Entities cooperate with each other.	Entities form bidirectional communication channels.	Outcomes: Broader health outcomes affecting broader community. Strong bidirectional trust built.
Outcomes: Optimally, establishes communication channels and channels for outreach.	Outcomes: Develops connections.	Outcomes: Visibility of partnership established with increased cooperation.	Outcomes: Partnership building, trust building.	

Source: Clinical and Translational Science Awards Consortium Community Engagement Key Function Committee Task Force. (2011). *Principles of community engagement* (2nd ed., p. 8). Washington, DC: US Government Printing Office. Retrieved from https://www.atsdr.cdc.gov/communityengagement/pdf/PCE_Report_508_FINAL.pdf

Level and Stage of Engagement

Although scientific methods remain as rigorous and require the same level of accountability as other grant applications, several things require more justification and explanation in a CE proposal. It should be apparent by now that writing a grant proposal for engaging communities requires some serious attention to the level of engagement your project proposes. In fact, the *level* of CE your grant proposes determines the extent to which specific elements of inclusion are required in the application. Often, the level of engagement depends on the stage of your engagement process. Although levels of engagement can vary from consultation to full participation, three levels and characteristics of engagement were described more explicitly in a document developed by the Access, Quality and Use in Reproductive Health (ACQUIRE) team called the *Active Community Engagement (ACE) Continuum*. The ACE Continuum was used to engage communities in reproductive health (RH) and family planning (FP) services through RH/FP programs.

> The continuum consists of three levels of engagement across five characteristics of engagement. The levels of engagement, which move from consultative to cooperative to collaborative, reflect the realities of RH/FP partnerships and programs. These three levels of community engagement can be adapted, with specific RH/FP inputs or activities based on these categories of action. The five characteristics of engagement are community involvement in assessment; access to information; inclusion in decision making; local capacity to advocate to institutions and governing structures; and accountability of institutions to the public. ACQUIRE's experience has shown that community engagement is not a one-time event, but rather is a process, and is an important consideration in the planning and evaluation of programs. (Russell, Igras, Johri, Kuoh, Pavin & Wickstrom, 2008, p. 2)

An important aspect in facilitating the engagement process is the ability to freely communicate with participants, orally and in written form. This may require skilled facilitators or navigators to avoid dominance by perceived elite groups (educators, physicians, social leaders) or to ensure that the language used is free from jargon or unfamiliar terms. An often underrecognized factor may be the unfamiliarity with the "culture" and the ways that language differs across groups. This is seen when dealing with diverse groups such as military, tribal, or clinical interest groups who have either governmental or social ownership of the problems and people you anticipate working with. Therefore it is crucial to begin with the problems and issues identified by the group in question. Sensitivity to how problem issues are shared with the public and in publications is an area that has scuttled projects in the past and, hence, should demand high attention from the outset. One place to begin is with a "round table" of people from each participatory group who are brought in as equals and with the opportunity to engage in open discussions. If permission is required from the top, as in governmental, organizational, or tribal groups, seek a knowledgeable navigator for assistance. Strengths of this approach are the assumption of equality, openness of discussion, focus on issues rather than people, and invitation for win-win solutions. Weaknesses pointed out from one group of experienced community planners in the United Kingdom include the lack of wider participation from academic or scientific professionals, the need for extensive preparation and highly skilled facilitators, and the potential for dominant professionals to intimidate lay or community participants (Community Places Team et al., 2014).

Importance of Trust

Building trust among academic, scientific, and community partners is identified as a crucial factor in overcoming collaborative barriers. Community members may have what some call "healthy paranoia" of researchers who are known to come, gather information, and then leave without making change (Horowitz et al., 2009). Likewise, there is often a similar barrier caused by the attitudes of researchers who fail to acknowledge the benefit that shared ideas brought from the community. These researchers often withhold information from the community. Without trust, the community will not give access to the research, and without accountability of researchers to the communities they study, there can be no trust. CE grant writing should be collaborative so that successful funding can be celebrated by the community members as "We got the grant" rather than "They got the grant" (Horowitz et al., 2009).

Involving a University or Institute in CE

Academic institutions and other large institutions with ongoing mechanisms for data management, review, and dissemination should prepare well in advance of individual project plans in discussions that involve potential funders. Whether there are governmental, tribal, academic, or scientific institutions among potential partners, it is reasonable to expect they will not all share the same fundamental culture, values, or regard for research information and its ownership. Frameworks have been developed for including CE in educating applicants and preparing peer reviewers (Ahmed & Palermo, 2010; Deverka et al., 2012). Several models of effective nonexploitive CE projects offer examples of how they were able to work through barriers to effective collaboration and are well worth reviewing in preparation for such a goal. In an early collaborative partnership to improve HIV prevention research, the investigators reported the importance of establishing an effective university–community–organization relationship to deal with barriers (Harper & Salina, 2000). Their principles are similar in scope and concerns to those being used a decade later. For example, Yale University CTSA'S Community Alliance for Research and Engagement (CARE), Ethical Principles of Engagement Committee added principles to include risks and benefits that could occur to one or more institutional partners, depending on study outcomes. They emphasize the importance of developing a "legitimate and serious dissemination plan" that includes (a) potential uses of all data to be collected, (b) plans for sharing data with the wider nonacademic community, and (c) a process for handling findings that may reflect negatively and thus cause harm to one or both partners (CARE Ethical Principles of Engagement Committee, 2009, p. 3).

Strategies for Meeting CE Grant Requirements

Recognizing that CE grants require a different approach, both applicant institutions and funding agencies have taken steps to train potential applicants. *Engagement* is defined by PCORI (2014) as "meaningful involvement of patients, caregivers, clinicians, and other healthcare stakeholders throughout the research process— from topic selection through design and conduct of research to dissemination of results." *Stakeholders* are "persons with current or past experience of illness or injury, family members or other unpaid caregivers of patients, or members of advocacy organizations that represent patients or caregivers" (PCORI, 2016). The underlying principle of stakeholder involvement has encouraged training programs to include community members as well as researchers and clinicians in the training. Each funding agency has strict requirements for the evidence of collaboration that should be included in the proposal. An excellent example of how well one research team complied with the requirements of a PCORI proposal mandates is apparent in their published research report (Ezenwa et al., 2017). PCORI set the bar for training and informing interested parties through their early "pipeline" efforts to seed new partnerships for new investigators (Selby & Lipstein, 2014). New investigators were invited to attend their regional meetings to explain the application process. Their well-defined "rubric" for what the grant proposal should contain (Sheridan et al., 2017) and their training booklet and resource guide are particularly explicit (PCORI, 2014).

CONCLUSION

Before you start a CE effort, think about the larger picture. By now, it should be clear that writing the grant proposal for CE funds is not the first step. In fact, the nine principles appearing in *Principles of Community Engagement*, 2nd ed. (CTSA, 2011), offer excellent guidelines for any CE effort (see Table 6.1). Take the time to learn from the experiences of others, including the recipients

TABLE 6.1

NINE UNDERLYING PRINCIPLES OF COMMUNITY ENGAGEMENT

Before you start a community engagement effort:

1. Be clear about the purposes or goals of the engagement effort and the populations and/or communities you want to engage with.
2. Become knowledgeable about the community's culture, economic conditions, social networks, political and power structures, norms and values, demographic trends, history, and experience with efforts by outside groups to engage it in various programs. Learn about the community's perceptions of those initiatives and the engagement activities.

For engagement to occur, these things are necessary:

1. Go to the community, establish relationships, build trust, work with the formal and informal leadership, and seek commitment from community organizations and leaders to create processes for mobilizing the community.
2. Remember and accept that collective self-determination is the responsibility and right of all people in a community. No external entity should assume it can bestow on a community the power to act in its own self-interest.

For engagement to succeed:

1. Partnering with the community is necessary to create change and improve health.
2. All aspects of community engagement must recognize and respect the diversity of the community. Awareness of the various cultures of a community and other factors affecting diversity must be paramount in planning, designing, and implementing approaches to engaging a community.
3. Community engagement can only be sustained by identifying and mobilizing community assets and strengths and by developing the community's capacity and resources to make decisions and take action.
4. Organizations that wish to engage a community as well as individuals seeking to effect changes must be prepared to release control of actions or interventions to the community and be flexible enough to meet its changing needs.
5. Community collaboration requires long-term commitment by the engaging organization and its partners.

Source: Clinical and Translational Science Awards Consortium Community Engagement Key Function Committee Task Force. (2011). *Principles of community engagement* (2nd ed., pp. 46–53). Washington, DC: US Government Printing Office. Retrieved from https://www.atsdr.cdc.gov/communityengagement/pdf/PCE_Report_508_FINAL.pdf

and funding agencies, about the benefits, barriers, and strategies that worked for them. When you are ready to engage your team of partners in grant writing, be attentive to the published requirements and follow them to the letter. Your proposal must reflect not only your knowledge and grantsmanship, but also the participation and commitment of all the partners. Your grant proposal must also show sensitivity to the original community needs in the evaluation plan, including not only the ways that objectives will be measured or met, but also the degree to which the community was engaged in the process.

REFERENCES

Ahmed, S. M., & Palermo, A.-G. S. (2010). Community engagement in research: Frameworks for education and peer review. *American Journal of Public Health, 100*(8), 1380–1387. doi:10.2105/AJPH.2009.178137

Centers for Disease Control and Prevention. (1997). *Principles of community engagement* (1st ed.). Atlanta, GA: CDC/ATSDR Committee on Community Engagement. Retrieved from https://www.atsdr.cdc.gov/communityengagement/pdf/PCE_Report_508_FINAL.pdf

Clinical and Translational Science Awards Consortium Community Engagement Key Function Committee Task Force. (2011). *Principles of community engagement* (2nd ed.). Washington, DC: US Government Printing Office. Retrieved from https://www.atsdr.cdc.gov/communityengagement/pdf/PCE_Report_508_FINAL.pdf

Community Alliance for Research and Engagement Ethical Principles of Engagement Committee. (2009). *Principles and guidelines for community-university research partnerships.* New Haven, CT: Yale University. Retrieved from https://depts.washington.edu/ccph/pdf_files/Principles_for_U-CPs_09-05-11_-_FINAL.pdf

Community Places Team, Bradley, C., O'Kane, L., Murtagh, B., Chanan, G., & Grarven, F. (2014). Community planning toolkit—Community engagement. Retrieved from http://www.communityplanningtoolkit.org/sites/default/files/Engagement.pdf

Deverka, P. A., Lavallee, D. C., Desai, P. J., Esmail, L. C., Ramsey, S. D., Veenstra, D. L., & Tunis, S. R. (2012). Stakeholder participation in comparative effectiveness research: Defining a framework for effective engagement. *Journal of Comparative Effectiveness Research, 1*(2), 181–194. doi:10.2217/cer.12.7

Ezenwa, M. O., Suarez, M. L., Carrasco, J. D., Hipp, T., Gill, A., Miller, J., … Wilkie, D. J. (2017). Implementing the PAIN RelieveIt randomized controlled trial in hospice care: Mechanisms for success and meeting PCORI methodology standards. *Western Journal of Nursing Research, 39*(7), 924–941. doi:10.1177/0193945916668328

Harper, G. W., & Salina, D. D. (2000). Building collaborative partnerships to improve community-based HIV prevention research: The University-CBO Collaborative Partnership (UCCP) model. *Journal of Prevention & Intervention in the Community, 19*(1), 1–20. doi:10.1300/J005v19n01_01

Holtzclaw, B. J. (2007). *Characteristics of a fundable research grant.* Paper presented at the Second Research Conference of the Association of Nurses in AIDS Care, San Antonio, TX.

Horowitz, C. R., Robinson, M., & Seifer, S. (2009). Community-based participatory research from the margin to the mainstream. *Circulation, 119*(19), 2633–2642. doi:10.1161/CIRCULATIONAHA.107.729863

Institute of Medicine. (2011). *Learning what works: Infrastructure required for comparative effectiveness research: workshop summary*. Washington, DC: The National Academies Press.

Israel, B., Schultz, A., Parker, E., Becker, A., Allen, A., III, & Guzman, R. (2008). Critical issues in developing and following CBPR principles. In M. Minkler & N. Wallerstein (Eds.), *Community-based participatory research for health: From process to outcomes* (2nd ed., pp. 47–66). San Francisco, CA: Jossey-Bass.

Israel, B., Schulz, A. J., Parker, E. A., & Becker, A. B.; Community-Campus Partnerships for Health. (2001). Community-based participatory research: Policy recommendations for promoting a partnership approach in health research. *Education for Health, 14*(2), 182–197. doi:10.1080/13576280110051055

National Academies of Sciences, Engineering, and Medicine. (2017). *Communities in action: Pathways to health equity*. Washington, DC: National Academies Press.

Patient-Centered Outcomes Research Institute. (2014). Methodology 101 training booklet and resource guide. Retrieved from https://www.pcori.org/sites/default/files/PCORI-Methodology-101-Training-Booklet-and-Resource-Guide.pdf

Patient-Centered Outcomes Research Institute. (2016). Patient-Centered Outcomes Research Institute: About us. Retrieved from http://www.pcori.org/about-us/our-programs

Russell, N., Igras, S., Johri, N., Kuoh, H., Pavin, M., & Wickstrom, J. (2008). The active community engagement continuum. ACQUIRE project working paper; USAID Cooperative Agreement No. GPO-A-00-03-00006-00. Retrieved from http://www.acquireproject.org/fileadmin/user_upload/ACQUIRE/Publications/ACE-Working-Paper-final.pdf

Selby, J. V., & Lipstein, S. H. (2014). PCORI at 3 years—progress, lessons, and plans. *New England Journal of Medicine, 370*(7), 592–595. doi:10.1056/NEJMp1313061

Sheridan, S., Schrandt, S., Forsythe, L., Hilliard, T. S., & Paez, K. A. (2017). The PCORI engagement rubric: Promising practices for partnering in research. *Annals of Family Medicine, 15*(2), 165–170. doi:10.1370/afm.2042

Talib, Z., Palsdottir, B., Briggs, M., Clithero, A., Miniclier Cobb, N., Marjadi, B., … Willems, S. (2017). Defining community-engaged health professional education: A step toward building the evidence. NAM Perspectives. Discussion Paper, National Academy of Medicine, Washington, DC. Retrieved from http://www.academia.edu/30742145/Defining_Community-Engaged_Health_Professional_Education_A_Step_Toward_Building_the_Evidence

7

. . .

Check Your Parachute! A Few More Hoops to Jump Through

. . .

GRANT JAIL: RECOGNIZING THE TIME COMMITMENT

Unless you have "been there and done that," you have no idea how time-consuming grant writing is. Like childbirth, many who have experienced it once tend to forget the downside or discomfort with the passage of time. Granted, most of us write grants in between other professional and family responsibilities. The reality is that at some point you must lock yourself up for a few hours or days to write and rewrite. It feels like grant jail! As the submission deadline gets nearer, numerous last-minute changes suggested or mandated by your institutional review board (IRB) or reviewers become necessary. This is when you cannot tolerate frequent interruptions if you plan to get the work done on schedule. Every change made in the grant may have ripple effects that make it necessary to make changes in the abstract, specific aims page, or methods. Failure to concentrate on the far-reaching effects of every revision leads to flaws in the overall application. Plan on setting aside some concentrated work time to finalize your proposal for submission. It may be only 1 or 2 hours, but devoting this time to the grant, if possible, will make a big difference in the outcome. Grant writing is not a quick process. Even short grants for foundations require a commitment of several days or weeks to write a tight, solid grant.

• • •

WHAT TO INCLUDE (OR NOT)

As you near the submission of your grant, revisit what should and should not be included with your packet. All grants are not the same, and even grants submitted to the same funding agency may require different documents for applications for different grant-funding mechanisms. The National Institutes of Health (NIH) is a good example of an agency that is progressively changing the items and configuration of pages required for a grant. A major change in NIH grant applications came when the itemized budget was eliminated from requested forms. Only a "consolidated" budget page is submitted to NIH on large grants. Streamlining of the award process has brought about "modular budgets" for new, competing continuation, and revised (amended) applications with budgets of $250,000 or less per year for direct costs; these budgets are for the following funding mechanisms:

- Research project grants (R01)
- Small grants (R03)
- Academic Research Enhancement Award (AREA) grants (R15)
- Exploratory/Development Research grants (R21)
- Clinical Trial Planning Grant Program (R34)
- Some Requests for Applications (RFAs) or Program Announcements (PAs)

Even though you may have figured dollars and cents on individual items, personnel, and equipment, the budget must conform to the modular amount allowed.

Pilot studies funded by NIH most often fall into the modular budget category to fund studies awarded no more than $100,000 for the complete project. An example of how funds are allocated can be seen in the R03 award. Applicants may request a project period of up to 2 years and a budget for direct costs of up to two $25,000 modules or one $50,000 module for a one-year grant. The NIH website (grants.nih.gov/grants) offers instruction on developing your budget and provides examples of completed forms. Enter "modular budgets" to explore instructions, frequently asked questions, and examples.

• • •

CHECK YOUR NIH PASSPORT: REQUIRED *eRA* REGISTRATION

Today's gateway to the NIH grant submission process is the *Electronic Research Administration (eRA) Commons* located at commons.era.nih.gov/commons. Designed to be an interface between the newer electronic submission process, reviewers, and applicants, the website provides access to information, grant application status, and all things of importance to NIH applicants and awardees. With the development of the eRA Commons, all applicants and applicant organizations must have a registration *username* and *password* to access the electronic submission process. You and your senior/key personnel must be registered to submit a grant proposal. If you have ever been registered with an eRA username and profile, you should maintain this single account throughout your career. An important reason to have a current eRA Commons account is that, since October 2007, grant review scores and feedback are available only through the web-based Commons. You must also be sure that your account is affiliated with any new institution if you move. Your signing official (SO) at your new location should be notified of your eRA information and can complete the process of establishing your new institutional affiliation. The SO is usually located in the office of sponsored research or office of research administration and has the institutional and legal authority to bind the institution in grant administration matters. As principal investigator (PI), you should be sure that your research team is also on board with eRA usernames, passwords, and current affiliations. If you are at a small institution that may be new to NIH applications, be sure that your institution is also registered. Most eligible institutions have already registered for a Commons registration, but if they have not, they must do so before you can submit your grant.

* * *

PACKAGING YOUR GRANT FOR SUBMISSION: OTHER REQUIRED FORMS

Depending on the size and complexity of your home institution and the requirements of the grant-funding agency to which you apply, the packaging and accompanying forms vary. If you have followed our advice, you have already looked into the need for approval by your supervising administrator and department by the time you are ready to submit your grant proposal. Equally important are the approvals required by the overall university, hospital, or health science center that will house your research grant. The awardee's institution, *not* the PI, becomes the *actual* grant recipient in most cases. In large institutions such as health science centers, the submitting center, college, or school may receive the funds, but the institution ensures and manages the award. As such, the institution assures grantors that they have met all the assurances and requirements of ethical and financial conduct in the management of awarded funds. When a grant is funded, the funding goes into institutional accounts and is allocated to the researcher only when requests match the specific budget details of the project.

Recognizing the great responsibility of institutions in managing large awards of research funding for numerous applicants from different sources makes the need for careful accounting, rigorous attention to ethical practices, and internal revenue processes beyond reproach. Violations or failure to comply could result in institutional censure, charges of scientific misconduct, and loss of present and future federal funding.

• • •

ASSURANCES AND CLEARANCES

It should be absolutely understood that your own particular grant proposal requires IRB (human subject or animal protection) clearances before any research can take place. What new researchers may not know are the important assurances and clearances that your university, school, or healthcare institution must pass as well. A close look at the grant application form will clue you into required specific assurance information and identification numbers that will necessitate a quick search. The best source of information about your particular institution's assurances, clearances, and internal requirements is your own office of research and contracts or research administration office. Many large institutions post these assurance documents and SO procedures on their institutional website.

Institutions receiving any federal funds are required to document that they have a formal human- and animal-protection committee that meets certain specifications for size and activities. Qualifying institutions are issued a human-subjects assurance number and an animal-welfare assurance number that must be included on the face page of federal grants. In addition, federal grants and most foundations require certification by the Internal Revenue Service of the institution's nonprofit status. This information is also required on the federal grant face page. There may be other assurances required by your institution, some of which may have already been filed, and for which there may exist a documented form.

Many institutions require an internal form to report disclosure of conflicts of interest in externally funded projects or external relationships and university activities. Another form may be required if the grant involves an employee jointly employed by two or more agencies (e.g., a person jointly employed by a university and a Veterans Administration agency). An internal memorandum of understanding must be filed prior to a grant submission to document that administration, clinical, research, and teaching activities add up to 100% of the person's total work activities. This serves to verify that no dual compensation for the same work is taking place and no actual or apparent conflict of commitment exists as well.

For federal grants, an *entity identifier* is used to identify each institution eligible for funding. This identifier contains the employer identification number assigned by the Internal Revenue Service, which is used for the submission of

Social Security and income-tax withholding payments. NIH grant applications require the entity identification number on the face page.

Since October 2003, federal grant applications or cooperative agreements have required institutions seeking grants to include a Dun & Bradstreet Data Universal Numbering System (D-U-N-S) number in every application for a new or competing continuation grant or cooperative agreement. There is a spot to enter your institution's DUNS number on every NIH grant application face page. If you are not associated directly with an institution that has a DUNS number, you can apply for one through Dun & Bradstreet. For example, if you have a consulting business, you or your business can apply for this number. Go to http://fedgov.dnb.com/webform

* * *

SHOWING RESEARCH PERSONNEL'S OTHER FUNDING

Listing your senior/key personnel's ongoing and completed grant funding is one way that your funding agency checks that there is no dual compensation for the same professional work or overlap of one grant's funding to another. This information previously appeared in NIH grants in a section called "Other Support." Today's NIH streamlined grant process calls for this information to be included on the last page of each person's biographical sketch under the heading of "Research Support and/or Scholastic Performance." In a prescribed format "Ongoing Research Support," as well as "Completed Research Support," is listed. Grants are listed with their grant number and mechanism, the name of the PI, the inclusive dates of the grant, the funding agency, the title, a brief one- or two-sentence description of the work, and the role of the applicant on the grant.

* * *

SPECIALLY REQUESTED TABLES

Although we have discussed the need for targeted enrollment tables for ethnic minorities, women, and children in federal research grants, there may be other requirements in training or demonstration grants for minority, graduation, or faculty tables. Tables showing faculty/student assignments, publication collaboration, and previous institutions of enrolled students enhance institutional training grants for doctoral study.

Tables for educational training grants present data on how many minority students are admitted to and have graduated from the institution submitting the grant. Graduation tables contain overall data on the number of students admitted and finally graduated from the various programs the school offers. Faculty tables are used by reviewers to see how many faculty are from ethnic minority groups, whether they are tenured, how many are full-time versus part-time, what the rank of each faculty member is, and what their areas of expertise are. These data help reviewers know if there are enough internal resources and individuals with the expertise specified in the grant to support the proposed program, special project, or research. These tables are usually not optional. Make sure they are included. Each section is given specific points, so missing tables detract from the overall points in the grant. It also suggests to the reviewers that the writer is unable to follow directions or is not detail oriented. Because tables occupy space in your grant and present a graphic representation of your program, take pains to have them constructed neatly by an experienced staff member. Review them carefully for errors and missing information.

* * *

DATA TO SUPPORT THE CASE FOR THE GRANT

Data to support the rationale for the research, practice, or educational grant must be detailed enough to let the reviewer know that the writer is aware of the national, regional, and local needs and healthcare trends. For example, if a cancer rehabilitation center is proposed, the rates and types of cancer in Denver may greatly differ from Chicago. This should be reflected in the writing. Data need to be current, and if no current data are available at one of these levels, then make sure to state that and why. Even an informal needs assessment strengthens the proposal. Include information on this assessment and the way that the data were collected. Giving only national data when the grant is administered locally is insufficient to provide a strong rationale for funding. Be as specific as you can in terms of each facet of the grant. Give accurate rationale to support your requests. Your grant should not appear to be adding to already adequate resources. Another important aspect is to project ongoing self-sufficiency. If the grant period is 3 years, how are you or your institution going to ensure that this program does not just die at the end of the funding cycle? The self-sufficiency statement, if requested, must be specific, with goals and acknowledgment of potential barriers. The potential barriers should have potential solutions built into the grant even though they are only projected. Not having a solid plan for sustainability can substantially reduce funding chances.

* * *

PRE-SUBMISSION REVIEW

The need for good presubmission review is so helpful to success that many nursing research centers build the process into their operation and hire experts to review grants before final submission. Some schools of nursing conduct mock reviews or "modeling parties" in which colleagues constructively critique grant applications to look for potential trouble spots. Hearing how discourse and discussion of a proposal can influence a group's scoring decision is helpful because this is exactly what a grant goes through at the funding agency. If getting a group together is not possible or if you fear your ability to tolerate honest feedback in a public forum, get one or more individuals to review your proposal privately. Try to decide who might be very objective but will give you good, constructive criticism that can improve your grant. Have these persons read the grant as if they were peer reviewers. They may be experts in the area of the grant and can make sure that you are quoting the most recent researchers or educators in the area (reviewers want to make sure you know your grant area and the key names associated with the grant's content area). Others might review the grant for flow and grammar and make sure that you have built a credible case for why it should be funded. Even if they have no knowledge of your grant area, they should be able to tell you if you have presented enough details to explain the rationale for the grant. An editor can also be extremely helpful in reviewing the grant by correcting grammar and cutting out excessive verbiage, formatting the application document, designing tables and figures, and checking references.

Presubmission reviewers may include some of the people in your institution who must read and sign off the grant prior to its submission. Their comments also help in the peer-review process. Of course, you will have to decide how many of the suggestions you will act on. The most important comments are those that reflect confusion about what you have written. Areas where your proposal has generated misunderstanding must be corrected. If reviewers have been part of previous grant-review panels, pay careful attention to their comments. They know what reviewers look for in grants and what constitutes a red flag.

* * *

AGENCY CONTACT PERSON FOR FINAL CHECKLIST OR TECHNICAL SUPPORT

As mentioned in earlier chapters, the contact person at your agency or technical support staff can be immensely helpful in the grant writing process. Draw on their expertise. They will help make sure your grant is complete. Use the checklist supplied with your application and, if included, the review criteria for the reviewers to ensure that all elements of the application are completed. Look at the criteria for selection and make sure your application addresses each of these points. Go over and over this checklist before you submit. Ideally, have someone else check the application with you; sometimes you cannot see your own omissions.

• • •

GRANT CHECKLIST

The grant checklist is the final step in the process. The NIH includes a checklist as part of the application. However, if your funding agency does not provide one, create your own consisting of each required element and the materials required by the agency. Review the checklist for submission again, and make sure that each item required is included in the packet. The checklist is part of the application packet. The list varies among funding agencies, but the basic elements are essentially the same. Look at the specific mailing instructions given in the packet. Grants mailed to the wrong person or the wrong addresses are often never reviewed. The person doing the electronic process checks off items on the checklist for the new SF242 electronic submission forms online. This may be your office of research administration.

• • •

GUIDELINES: READ, REREAD, AND PRAY!

Just as with the checklist, go over the actual guidelines for the grant. Review the funding areas, and the key words or objectives that the application packet uses; use these terms as headers and descriptors in your grant. It shows the reviewers that you read and paid attention to details. If you make a change in one section of the grant, make sure that the table or other sections also contain this information as well. Depending on the type of grant you are submitting or the type of institution in which you are working, determine whether optional tables or sections are needed. These are small items that are often overlooked in the grant. If someone else is copying and compiling multiple files to create your grant, make sure the final copies include all the pages in the order you want them. Omission of pages or paragraphs can make the grant incomplete and sometimes invalid for review. Be sure to scan or photocopy pages with signatures to be submitted as portable document format (PDF) files. This compiled version of your grant may need a final internal review by your institutional supervisor, dean, or director before it can be sent to your office of research administration for submission. Once you have done your best to review these items, have reviewed the guidelines, and have checked everything on the application checklist, begin the submission process, sit back, and pray.

CONCLUSION

A well-planned submission process makes grant writing much easier. The key is to plan, plan, and plan. Be realistic in your timeline for completion. Dedicate time to the actual writing *and* editing of the project. Have it reviewed by others not involved in the grant, and be ready to revise your proposal if revision is warranted. On the rare occasion when you are required to mail a proposal, be sure to check the final pages to be sure they have all been copied, printed, and numbered. Be sure to reexamine your grant proposal checklist just before the grant is mailed.

8

• • •

The Electronic Environment
of Grantsmanship

• • •

INTERNET CONNECTIONS TO YOUR GRANT SUBMISSION PORTAL

The rapid rise of electronic technology in the past three decades has affected grant writing in significant ways. From the efficient use of access to online literature to support a research proposal to the word-processing ease the computer provides, a researcher must be computer-savvy and able to connect with Internet resources. Your research team must have investigators and staff who can communicate and interact with electronic systems. Today's electronic grant submission platforms are required by federal, foundation, commercial, and academic funding sources. Even some small organizations or chapters have moved to online drop box systems for grant applications. The Internet is your channel for grant information, and for communication with local, institutional, and global resources, you will need to submit, process, review, and report grant documents.

• • •

PREPARING FOR AN ELECTRONIC FLIGHT

Writing the proposal for electronic transmission requires a few different approaches from the old method of fitting text to a page. Instead, the newer requirements are not sized to the page until they are "dropped" into specific blocks on computerized forms. Some form blocks have word counts or lines of text prescribed, whereas others are mandated to numbers of pages. The National Institutes of Health (NIH) has such a variety of grants and forms, and it helps to take advantage of the evolving NIH-specific training offered online. The full array of training can be accessed at grants.nih.gov/grants/about_grants.htm, and a four-part tutorial on writing the NIH grant is described at grants.nih.gov/grants/how-to-apply-application-guide/video/prepare-to-apply/index.htm on YouTube. Because websites change, additions or changes to the NIH training should be accessible at www.nih.gov.

Be sure to select the correct application instructions for your grant proposal. The NIH has five general types of grant forms: Research (R), Career Development (K), Training (T), Multi-Project (M), and Small Business (B). The NIH has specific training modules that give you the page limits for different types or funding mechanisms of grants (R, K, T, M, and B awards of varying types). They also warn you to check the specific Funding Opportunity Announcement (FOA) for page limits because they supersede the general page limits.

• • •

CHECK OUT THE eRA COMMONS' EXPANDED ELECTRONIC ENVIRONMENT

What Is the eRA?

The NIH completed its major update to its portal to electronic services, the Electronic Research Administration (eRA) Commons, in 2007. Since then, the eRA Commons has become the hub of all grant-related things and a virtual meeting place for the exchange of health-related research information from NIH extramural recipient organizations, grant awardees, and public members. The eRA written narratives have been vastly expanded and improved by integrating them with diagrams and flowcharts. YouTube links take you to videos that clearly explain the steps necessary to register for an eRA account and prepare, format, and submit a proposal. Specific YouTube videos explain different funding mechanisms and applications. The eRA website provides information on training, modules and user guides on eRA resources, rosters of NIH Scientific Review Groups, and links to major federal funding sources that fund training and project grants, such as NIH'S Office of Extramural Research (OER), the Agency for Healthcare Research and Quality (AHRQ), the Centers for Disease Control and Prevention (CDC), the Food and Drug Administration (FDA), and the Substance Abuse and Mental Health Services Administration (SAMHSA). Accessed at public.era.nih.gov/commons, helpful links include the steps of the electronic application process, a demonstration of what the eRA Commons offers, training events, and specific help buttons. The eRA Commons has both unrestricted and restricted areas that allow free access for public information and controlled access for confidential information. Among the training features are videos that include guides to getting registered, use of the forms, use of the status feature to see where your grant proposal is in the review chain, and explanations of the many processes used by federal grant agencies.

Your eRA Account Is a Necessity!

You must be registered with eRA to submit a federal grant, and becoming registered offers you the fullest access to eRA resources as you develop your proposal. Registering lets you set up an account name to be used throughout your career. Your user name must be unique within the eRA Commons community and is affiliated with your initial place of employment. If you move to a new institution, your new research administration must change your affiliating institution. Your eRA username also appears on your biographical sketch that accompanies your proposal, as well as someone else's grant that includes your participation.

A major advantage of having a restricted account is the ability to view the status of your grant proposal as it goes through the committee review process. Your institution's research grant administrator can also access your grant status, see a summary view of grant applications, review the Notice of Grant Award, and access the Progress Report face page. This feature is helpful if you have questions about any of the postings and their meanings. The old familiar written notification of grant award (still called a "pink sheet" by some, even though it has not actually been pink for decades) has been replaced by electronic notification. The NIH has not provided paper notification of the Notice of Award letters since 2007. Instead, notices are sent solely via email to grantee organizations and are accessible in the eRA Commons. This means that feedback is received when it is posted and you do not have to wait for the form to be printed and mailed. You will receive the Notice of Grant Award through the eRA Commons Status Module. Once a grant has been awarded to you, your annual progress report of accomplishments and award compliances will be documented by you in the research performance progress report (RPPR) and submitted online. At the end of your grant period, the final progress report (FPR) is filed for the grant closeout.

Other benefits offered by the NIH eRA process are an easier compilation process for the applicant. Page numbers and the table of contents are system generated and included in the final grant application. Because the sections of your grant proposal are done automatically, the system paginates your proposal and generates a customized table of contents on the basis of your specific submission. Any nonrelevant items that formerly appeared on the older standardized pages no longer appear.

NIH electronic submission also has advantages for grant reviewers who are able to access and download the grants and materials on the eRA Commons, view and use computerized search features, and carry their laptop instead of stacks of proposals to study section review meetings. The Internet-assisted review (IAR) process allows reviewers to submit critiques and preliminary scores for applications they are reviewing without having to worry about mails or emails arriving at their destination.

• • •

ELECTRONIC FLIGHT PLAN FOR GRANT SUBMISSION

Given the potential for saving costs in mailing, communication, and paper, it is not surprising that the federal government was an early adopter for electronic submission of grant proposals. The NIH expected that getting rid of paper copies would eliminate approximately 200 million pieces of paper a year and reduce the costs of scanning, data entry, data validation, printing, and reproduction. The NIH rolled out its electronic submission process in 2005 with the Small Business Innovative Research (SBIR) and Small Business Technology Transfer Program (STTR) grant proposals. Other federal agencies such as the Health Resources & Services Administration (HRSA) and the AHRQ followed suit. The electronic transition of all federal grant submissions has taken place at every level, and many foundation grants have also followed suit.

• • •

CYBER-SUBMISSION? IS THIS TRIP NECESSARY?

As with all new things, those involved with the process met the prospect of online submission with varying degrees of enthusiasm, delight, distress, and disgust. Potential grant applicants and their research administration offices shared anxieties about the process, access, and time needed for submission. Their primary fear was that the electronic process would be difficult and require excessive training. Grant reviewers accustomed to receiving paper copies fretted about whether they would be able to find an electronic copy legible. This fear was prompted in part by the NIH'S simultaneous move away from its old familiar PHS398 application form to the SF424 Research and Related (R&R) form for all its electronic submissions. Instead of compiling a single document as in the past, the new electronic grant is built by filling out electronic forms by cutting and pasting grant proposals, created with a computer's word-processing program, into the template form. A cautionary word is that you should not try to fill out these online forms without thoroughly reviewing your work for errors or omissions. You need to carefully refine what is placed in the form, and you may need to become more succinct to meet space limits. This ensures that you put your best document and profile of your work forward. Fortunately, there is no longer a need to have special software for creating the proposal text, and NIH provides a link for free download of software to convert letters and reprints into portable document format (PDF) files for online submission.

Ever-evolving changes made it necessary for applicants to tune into the funding agency to keep up with the changes, the priorities, and even the language encouraged for success. With proactive administrative help from institutions, the process in most cases has not been formidable, and help from the funding agency has been expanded. The NIH was anticipatory in making available free workshops and step-by-step procedures from its website to help alleviate fears and prepare institutional grant offices. Although there were a few complaints from reviewers who disliked reviewing grant proposals on a computer and objected to printing out their own copies, the transition to electronic submissions was not as bad as expected. Other funding agencies, including the American Nurses Foundation (ANF), the Robert Wood Johnson Foundation (RWJF), Sigma Theta Tau International (STTI), and the regional research societies have joined the trend toward electronic proposals. Gone are the stacks of bulky proposals, the late-night trips to the FedEx office, and anxieties about ground mail delivery. In their place are new mandates for planning ahead and timely submissions to institutional grant offices for sign-offs. Scenarios that involve staying up all night to complete a grant proposal and hand-carrying it by plane to Washington on its due date are obsolete. You must recognize that grant proposals are now processed in an electronic environment. Be sure that you are on board and have electronic navigators to help you. This may be your research administration office, your technology staff, or a knowledgeable administrative assistant. Get help early and plan for your learning curve. Take advantage of institutional workshops and online training about electronic grant submission. Familiarity with the language, rules, and processes makes it less confusing. Remember that many of the rules and information details are evolving. Look for the most recent versions of instructions, and be ready to encounter a few bumps in the journey. You can do this, and there is help available to you along the way.

· · ·

GENERAL RULES FOR ELECTRONIC SUBMISSION

- **Strive for error-free originals:** Submitting any type of grant application online requires the development of error-free originals. Use your computer's word-processing software to type your budget pages, biographical sketches, and research plan on paper forms first, then print them out, and proofread carefully. Spell-check features in your word-processing program are helpful, but watch out for words that sound the same but have different meanings that are misused (the most common error is in using "principle investigator" when you mean "principal investigator"). Enlist at least one other person to follow behind you on your check for errors or missing items.

- **Watch software, format, and space issues:** Old estimates about numbers of pages or words per page may not apply when document submissions are online. Be sure to check the guidelines and regulations at the submission website and use the recommended format and headings if they are given. Double-check to see what font is recommended and whether documents are single or double spaced. Check out the application website to be sure you are using the appropriate version of a word-processing program for online submissions. For NIH grants, the currrent recommended software for downloading, completing, and submitting NIH forms is Adobe Acrobat Reader for Windows or MAC and more information is available online from the Grants.gov website. Compatible versions of Adobe Reader software may be found on Grant.gov's Adobe Software Compatibility page and are needed to view PDF documents, including the application images assembled by eRA systems.

- **Use a citation manager with your electronic proposal submission:** A citation manager, such as EndNote (Carlsbad, CA: Thompson ResearchSoft), ProCite (Carlsbad, CA: Thompson ResearchSoft), or Reference Manager (Carlsbad, CA: Thompson ResearchSoft), can be a benefit in grant writing. To save precious space in the narrative, superscripted numbers are often used as citations instead of lengthy names and years. The tedious process of referencing citations is facilitated by modern citation managers that automatically type them in order of appearance in the grant proposal. Be aware, however, that these references are coded by the citation software and can become jumbled when they are moved from one platform to another. One way to avoid this is to remove the citation manager codes from the final copy by converting the document to plain text. This keeps all the citations and the reference list in place but no longer active with the citation manager. Just be sure to keep a copy with all the citation manager codes intact in case you have to return to the application and revise.

- **Check the source for updates and changes:** The NIH website and support facilities rapidly change, both in process and in name. Each year the guidelines for NIH grant applications undergo changes that make it imperative to *check the source* for new and evolving updates. How NIH grants are submitted varies with your organization's rules, so check with your administrative or grants management office to see if you or the institution will prepare and submit application data to the Grant.gov website. Submission requirements and presubmission regulations of the NIH make institution-to-institution grant submission less challenging for the investigator without an administrative infrastructure. The NIH "How to Apply" link offers detailed information for the preparation, submission, and tracking of grant applications. Guidelines are offered at https://grants.nih.gov/grants/how-to-apply-application-guide.html. Other funding agencies may have moved from paper submission to partial online submission, with letters and signed documents mailed as paper files. More recently, it has become common for signed documents to be submitted as PDF files sent electronically.

- **Get permission to apply:** Plan if your grant application needs institutional or funder approval before you can apply. Highly competitive grants or center grants may be limited by the funding agency or by your institution to one application submission in the current grant cycle. The RWJF and the National Palliative Care Research Center (NPCRC) streamline their selection and review process by asking for abbreviated documents such as a letter of intent or a "miniproposal" to help screen proposals. Full proposals "are accepted by invitation only." Some funding agencies only allow one application to be submitted from a single institution or university. For example, the Nurse Education, Practice, and Retention (NEPR) program funded by the HRSA has nine purposes, but an applicant organization may submit only one application per NEPR purpose under this announcement.

- **Register in eRA Commons:** The principal investigator and key personnel should all be registered in the eRA Commons and have usernames and passwords well in advance of an NIH grant submission. Registration can take several weeks to process, and you cannot submit an electronic federal grant without these numbers. Your office of research administration is the best resource to help you obtain this registration. Your Commons account follows you throughout your career, even if you move to another institution. Also, if you become an NIH consultant or grant reviewer, you keep the same Commons account and username. Likewise, grant reviewers who acquire a Commons account and username during that activity use the same registration, account, and username to submit a federal grant.

- **Ensure your organization's eRA Commons registration:** All applicant organizations need to be registered in Grants.gov and the eRA Commons well in advance of the submission date and before you can submit an electronic federal grant. Any organization applying for registration must also supply taxpayer identification number, Dun & Bradstreet Data Universal Numbering System (D-U-N-S), and Internal Revenue Service clearances, all of which can take considerable time. Your office of research administration or grants office should be able to provide you with the institutional eRA Commons username. If you are not sure whether the organization where you are a student, faculty member, or employee has a contracts office, contact your top administrative office early. Other detailed information about registration appears at the eRA Commons website at public.era.nih.gov/commons.

- **Use other points of reference for electronic searches:**
  - eRA Commons (public.era.nih.gov/commons) provides information technology solutions and support virtually for the full life cycle of grants administration functions for the NIH, operating divisions of the U.S. Department of Health and Human Services, and other federal agencies.
  - Grants.gov (Grants.gov) is the electronic source to find and apply for federal government grants.
  - HRSA (www.hrsa.gov) is an agency of the U.S. Department of Health and Human Services with a mission to improve access to healthcare services for people who are uninsured, isolated, or medically vulnerable. Grant pages at www.hrsa.gov/grants/index.html offer information on numerous funding opportunities in providing healthcare services for underserved people and for nursing and health professions training at several levels.
  - The NIH (www.nih.gov) offers access to all NIH institutes and centers, training resources, research funding, initiatives, NIH employment, and publications. Websites for specific institutes that fund pilot and major studies can be accessed from this site or from their own website addresses (e.g., National Institute of Nursing Research at www.ninr .nih.gov, National Institute on Aging at www.nia.nih.gov).

• • •

KEEPING A PAPER TRAIL IN A PAPERLESS ENVIRONMENT

Submitting grant proposals, or pieces of proposals, online tends to make researchers feel a bit fragmented. In fact, with NIH submissions, your proposal does not "come together" until the application data go through the Grants.gov submission and the eRA system compiles the data fields and attachments into a single grant application. At this time, applicants can see the entire grant application for the first time in the eRA Commons. If your application had validation or missing identifiers and did not make it through the eRA Commons application checking process, you must correct any errors and submit a corrected application to Grants. gov before your application can proceed further. If you had omitted something that was essential to your proposal, it might not be picked for review. Check with your NIH science officer to determine whether the missing element can be added or whether it requires submission of an entire corrected application.

With small foundation or professional organization grant applications, you could find that you do not have a complete copy of your document unless you take precautions to print or electronically save each page you submit. It is in your best interest to have a complete copy to refer to during and after your grant proposal has been reviewed. Print each screen before you submit the sections. Keeping a loose-leaf notebook with sections matching each grant section allows you to develop your paper copy as you submit pages. This notebook makes it easy to refer to sections if or when a funding agency calls you for specific information about your grant proposal. Knowing what you submitted is key to keeping track of your commitments and obligations. It provides a framework for ongoing reports when a grant is finally funded.

If your grant administration office is submitting your online foundation or organizational grant, ask it to provide a paper copy. Keep this copy in your loose-leaf notebook. NIH submissions produce a PDF copy of the compiled grant that your grant administration office will make available to you. This compiled copy will also be what your grant review committee finally reviews. It is important that you examine it closely to be sure that you have included everything you intended. A trail of forgotten pages, letters, consent forms, and other missing items makes it clear that these errors are common. However, it is in your best interest to find such omissions early enough to correct them *before* they are found in review.

CONCLUSION

Electronic grant submissions are here to stay, with foundations and professional organizations following the lead of federal funding agencies in adopting them. These technological changes offer new advantages, including an online view of your grant status and final feedback. The new set of skills required to function in an electronic environment is not rocket science, but advances in technology spur change. Keep in touch with changing organizations, forms, and processes. Take them step by step, seek help when you need it, and enjoy their advantages.

9

Gauging Progress
and Reviewer Feedback

THE ENVELOPE, PLEASE!

The results of your grant applications no longer are sent on "pink sheets"; however, they still hold the same weight. We still feel that they are either ego busters or ego boosters. Whether the notification of your grant status comes in an envelope, email, or a website posting, the excitement and anxiety are palpable. In earlier days, some of us who received notification by mail at work would go into a restroom stall to read it. The results that followed were unpredictable. If the envelope held a grant score, the applicant often emerged puzzled and had to seek more information as to its meaning from a senior researcher. If the message was congratulatory, the bathroom trip was short, and we all soon shared in celebration. If the trip was prolonged, it likely meant that the message was disappointing, and we felt empathy amid tears and tissues. Disappointment should not be misinterpreted as failure. Even the experienced grant writer experiences disappointments and successes in proposal writing.

BEHOLD THE TURTLE!

A wise research mentor once shared an analogy that is true to the task of a successful grant applicant. "Behold the noble turtle. To get ahead he has to stick his neck out and carry a hard shell." The image of daring to enter the race, slow persistence, and the ability to take the critique process without feeling a personal affront are characteristics that keep a researcher on the path to success. Part of our difficulty comes from the love/hate relationship we have with reviews or evaluations of any kind. We can't wait to get feedback on our grant application and are dying to know if we were funded, but we also have an awful dread of hearing any possibility that we weren't. This same dread of criticism tends to make us sidestep much-needed presubmission reviews or avoid mock study sections of our grant proposal in the first place. We quickly learn that it is crucial to develop a tough spine or some insensitivity to the process.

• • •

REVIEWERS ARE EXPERTS, BUT THEY ARE HUMAN

Bear in mind that the grant reviewers are enlisted to read and critique your proposal. They are often paid, or at least rewarded in some way for doing this, although seldom enough to truly pay for the time and effort they devote to the task. Because much is expected of the reviewers, they generally take great pains to do a thorough job and find errors and inconsistencies you may have overlooked. The National Institutes of Health (NIH) or Health Resources & Services Administration (HRSA) reviewers, for example, also write a narrative summary listing the strengths, weaknesses, and any changes they recommend. Because they are experts, they often go to great lengths to explain in detail where you have gone wrong. Contrary to what the applicant may feel, reviewers are not out to reject your proposal, they like nothing better than to find proposals that meet all the criteria for funding. On the other hand, they are not chosen to overlook shortcomings in a proposal, no matter how well intentioned. They also have low tolerance for sloppily written or submitted proposals. The fear is that this is the way you would conduct the project as well. Another factor to remember is the likelihood that your grant proposal was discussed in a group of several reviewers, so both positive and negative remarks in the critical review have likely influenced the final review summary you receive. Often, review of a proposal deemed highly acceptable by one reviewer will be dampened by that of another. This can happen in the other direction as well. One reviewer may have a hard time finding any redeeming features in a proposal but will change their mind when hearing the positive attributes found by another reviewer. All reviewers are reasonable human beings, and although they are experts with skills in reviewing, they hold subjective biases and opinions. They must come to an agreement to score or approve your proposal, so the final score is often a compromise among reviewers. If the review was positive and they thought your grant proposal was innovative and wonderful, you're entitled to a huge ego boost. If it is clear that the comments are universally negative, allow yourself a brief pity party, then get back to work. The following tips are shared here to help you better understand and get the most out of reviewer feedback and use it to move forward. Begin by reading the review carefully, taking notes and highlighting the comments. Then begin translating what the review is really trying to tell you. Also remember, if this is a review of a resubmission, you may in fact receive a far different review from the first. This difference may be due to the change in composition of the reviewers or the landscape could have changed in your area since your previous submission. For example, the first year that bioterrorism grants were requested there was a "hunger" for these grants. But 2 to 3 years later, the science and educational strategies had advanced so just a simple resubmission of a rejected grant during the first year, 2 or 3 years later would have to be significantly more sophisticated. These factors make it usually advantageous to plan resubmissions as soon as feasible to keep up with the shifting landscape.

● ● ●

TRANSLATING THE REVIEW

Grant proposal reviews tend to fall into four categories: reviews that say:

1. Yes, we love your proposal as it is.
2. Yes, this is acceptable with a few simple additions or revisions.
3. Possibly, in a resubmission with extensive revisions.
4. No, this isn't going to meet our needs, priorities, or standards.

The first category is fairly straightforward, and you may need to pinch yourself to be sure you fully understand that "yes, you've been funded!" The second category may refer to some hoops you need to jump through, questions you need to answer, or documents you need to supply before funding can be ensured. Category three and four are the hardest to decipher, especially if your results say that your study has been "approved, but not funded." Some foundations are likely to say that if it is a dissertation or thesis project, to not discourage a student whose work had already been approved by their university committee. However, sometimes a granting agency approves a project on its merit but does not have sufficient funds to award all their meritorious applications. If this is the case with regard to your grant proposal, it should encourage you to seek another funder. Some applicants look for clues in their NIH or HRSA scoring to determine which category their review falls in, but this is not a reliable indicator. Excellent ideas are sometimes given less competitive scores if there is a clear omission of an important section, resource, or support. Look at the comments as indicators of whether it is your idea or the way it is implemented that has prompted your reviewers' response. On the other hand, a score that is near the top of the scoring range probably has fewer things that need to be revised for a resubmission. Scoring ranges for NIH reviews are from 1 (exceptional) to 9 (poor), whereas HRSA grants are scored in percentages with 100% as outstanding and 59% or lower as poor.

• • •

WHAT YOU CAN LEARN

Try to interpret the meaning of the reviewers' message in light of your proposal. Did you feel a time crunch to submit the grant proposal before you had all the details worked out? Did the reviewers cast doubt on your abilities to carry out the project? Were you lacking a working team or resources to carry out the planned activities? These comments give you a fairly clear direction for resubmission, and you will know where you need to spend your efforts for resubmission. Have the reviewers failed to understand what you had in mind? In this case, it may be that your writing skills need help and that you need technical assistance in the mechanics of grant writing. Making your idea more understandable is something a writing consultant can help you with. Most academic and hospital settings provide resources to assist with the grant writing process. Commercial programs are also available that provide proposal master templates that help guide the grant writer through the process.

Do the reviewers express doubt that your idea will work? Pilot studies are the strongest evidence that an idea is workable or a phenomenon is measurable. In fact, some researchers carry out small pilot studies to address this issue while waiting for grants to be reviewed. Was there insufficient evidence that the problem, significance, or relevance was worthy of grant support? These comments require a more convincing argument that the problem is of concern and relevance to the funding agency. Less clear are comments that cast doubts on your ideas. Unfortunately, this is the area in which most grant applications are scored down in the review process. The idea itself may be something you are so close to and passionate about that you cannot be objective about its importance or significance. If your interpretation of the review is that the idea didn't measure up, engage an honest expert to level with you about its weaknesses and strengths. This needs to be not only a person you trust, but also someone knowledgeable about your scientific or scholarship area. Perhaps it is an idea whose time has not yet come. If that is the case, you can tuck it away in your treasure box and proceed to build some preliminary work that may show its relevance or replace it with a better idea.

Sometimes, you are urged to submit an ill-prepared grant proposal to meet the needs of employing institutions. It may be that you had to submit the grant proposal too quickly or too early in the process. For example, educators are sometimes forced, due to budget restraints, to submit a program grant well before the "idea" is really ready. At times, your institution includes barriers, such as courses that have little relevance to your proposed program but have been required by the system for decades. In such a case, harsh reviewers' comments may provide impetus for institutional change. So, at your ego's expense you may have become a change agent!

Look to see if there is a hidden agenda in the review; perhaps the slant you took on the funding priority is not congruent with what the foundation was looking for at this time. Perhaps the grant reviewers' comments were influenced by their own areas of expertise. You may have missed subtle cues in their application kit that could be addressed if you are given the opportunity to resubmit. If it is a foundation grant with a small budget, it may be that your grant was one of many well-written proposals, so there wasn't enough money to fund them all. In this way, even a rejection may not mean that you wrote a bad grant proposal, although it will certainly feel that way at first. If it is an NIH or other federal grant involving a two-tier review, the scoring is done on merit and grant criteria without regard to the funding budget. In this case, the reviewer comments are your best clue to the ultimate decision.

• • •

DEVELOPING A POSITIVE APPROACH TO CRITIQUE

You have led a sheltered life if you have not experienced disappointment or rejection of a prized idea. Remembering that grants are proposals, and that you are among many suitors, helps you develop a positive philosophy toward critique as a conditioning technique. Like any other learned pursuit, the more it is practiced, the better the performances. One must therefore decide how to respond to critical review and practice it along the way. Here are some tips to guide you:

- **Expect alterations and revisions:** Do not fall into the trap of falling in love with your written words, but write and revise paragraphs often. See how many extraneous words you can remove but still be clear. This is called "crisping" your proposal.
- **Be prepared to submit a revised proposal:** It is a good idea to be prepared for the possible event of not being funded the first time around. Many grant proposals have repeat submission cycles that allow you to revise and resubmit in a timely manner. Revisions of projects with good ideas generally have a better chance as resubmissions than simply turning to a different funding agency. The amended proposal allows you to show how responsive you have been to reviewer's comments. If you submit to a different agency, you are starting over again; it is not like resubmitting to the same agency. Prolonging your time to resubmission may put you

in the same situation. The new review committee may have a whole new list of concerns about your proposal.

- **The more you write, the easier it gets:** It is hard for some people to believe that something hard gets easier when you keep doing it, but for the most part those who feel this way about writing are dealing with fear of failure. The beauty of computers is that you can write and write and never waste any paper. Set aside time to write, and then polish your writing. Tools such as a thesaurus, spellchecker, or grammatical program are available as computer aids. Taking a course in scientific writing can be helpful for those who tend to write copious prose or inverted sentences. Unlike a novel that holds the answer at the end, scientific writing needs to convey the idea up front and elaborate later.

- **Avoid getting wedded to your own words:** Unwillingness to give up a hard-earned paragraph is a symptom of those who struggle to write. Write it, using the Track Changes feature (in Microsoft Word) to make it better. If you think a phrase is "precious" and you are up against those suggesting that it is inflated or pretentious, print it out on a piece of paper and put it in your jewelry box. You might use it later.

- **Invite review and critique of your work:** Finding someone who is willing to read and objectively critique your work is a gift worth millions. Oddly enough, most academic settings have mentors or experts that are willing to do that voluntarily. If none are available to you, then push for your employing agency to hire consultants for this purpose. Often, retired faculty members are willing to do this type of consultation. On a much easier level, get together a group of colleagues who are in the same boat. Form a review group to go over one another's proposals or writing. Make a pact to give constructive criticism (it will be of no use to you if you only praise one another). Remember, this is "conditioning" critique to better prepare you for the real show!

- **Build on reviewer comments:** Consider every comment as important. Reviewer comments are the only clues you have for evaluating the strength of your proposal. To build on positive comments, try to determine the difference between enthusiastic comments and faint praise that the reviewer used to balance "strengths" with all of the weaknesses. Map out the "weakness" comments so that you fully understand what was missing, undersupported, or a bad idea. Not all foundations give you a detailed review of your grant proposal and nothing is less helpful than a rejected grant proposal with little or no feedback. If your grant proposal is rejected from a funding agency with little feedback, consult a faculty member who is an experienced grant writer before you resubmit your proposal.

- **Dealing with rejected grant submissions:** If you are going to write grant proposals, you will undoubtedly deal at some point with rejection.

Submissions at the federal level often take three to four submissions of the same grant before it is funded. Out-and-out rejection is disappointing. Always remember, it was your *proposal*, not *you*, that was rejected. The proposal can be revised, even thrown out if you find it cannot be repaired, but you are now wiser and more experienced in grant writing than you were before. You have joined the ranks of experienced grant writers who know that this is an expected rough patch that you can move through. Regard the review process as a learning experience. If the review was extremely harsh, put it away for a while and then go back when you are ready to really read the comments instead of reacting to them. "Try, try again," must be your motto.

• • •

SUBMITTING AN AMENDED PROPOSAL

A revised grant application (now called an "amended" application by NIH) is one that is resubmitted to the same funding agency. Federal grants, such as NIH, require an "introduction" to explain to the reviewers how you have addressed the previous critique. Carefully address specific comments and weaknesses pointed out in the earlier review and explain generally how you have corrected them. You are expected by NIH to amend the earlier application by using a different font feature (italicizing, underlining, or bolding) for any new additions or replacements. Because you replace unwanted text with the amended text, explain in your introduction which feature you are using to show changes. Your introduction should be respectful, not argumentative. Sarcasm immediately turns off your reviewers. If you decide that an aspect of your prior submission should stay in the proposal despite recommendations to remove it, respectfully provide new, stronger rationale and support for its inclusion. Experts have told you to make a change, so be sure that your new argument is convincing. The funding agency gives instructions in their guide to revisions about how much space you are allowed for an introduction or explanation.

CONCLUSION

The dreaded grant proposal's review results and summary provide a great deal of good information. The comments, if specific enough, can help you refine your grant proposal even if it was funded. If the grant was not funded, use the comments to revise the grant proposal for resubmission to the same funding agency or to another one that might be more appropriate. If you have received funding, your work has just begun! The next chapter will offer some tips for your journey.

10

So Now You've Been Funded

GLOW OF SUCCESS!

Congratulations! What an accomplishment a funded research study is. You are finally out of grant jail! Take some time to bask in that reality when it happens. You earned it! Okay, take maybe one day, but then wake up and smell the coffee. This is when your work really begins. What will you do next? You will benefit by acknowledging some important facts to make your newly funded grant successful and enjoyable to all its participants. Probably the most important fact is that carrying out the research *takes time*. You need to carve out that time as if it were a job. If your grant includes some salary support, arranging time for the study is much easier. If it does not, you must either negotiate the time to carry your project out from your regular employment or find time above and beyond your workday. We have dedicated this chapter to the importance of getting a grip on your time, organizing your work, and avoiding some common pitfalls in carrying out your work. Planning in the grant proposal for what needs to be done, and in what order, makes this step easier after you receive funding.

DUST OFF THAT TIMELINE

Do you recall the timeline we discussed in Chapter 5? What might have been a skeleton plan for your proposal now becomes your map for action. This is the time to flesh it out with activities, dates, and assignments. Add dates for submitting annual reports, meeting with your team, and updating your institutional review board (IRB) reports. Enlarge and keep your timeline posted in a conspicuous place. Some items can be modified, whereas others are less flexible. Without a timeline, you are like a navigator without a map or GPS.

* * *

TIME TO GET ORGANIZED!

Many principal investigators (PIs) and project directors find a way to "bind" the project together. One simple way to do this is to begin putting documents in a three-ring binder or an electronic secured file folder (this is especially nice if it is cloud-based and accessible at work and home) from the time you submit the grant to the end of the project. Use dividers with labels or different file folders to separate sections of your proposal into those dealing with budget and those focused on the project itself. This makes it easy to refer to the road map for the project and to keep the integrity of the plan intact. It is also useful if someone from the funding budget office or your own research administration office calls and needs some data from the original submission. Once the grant is funded, make a photocopy or an electronic copy of the funding notice for your notebook/folder and label that. It provides you with your grant number, the actual dollars funded, and other information you may need later. The notebook or folder can contain a section for correspondence about the grant between you, your funding agency, your consultants, and your clinical or community sites. Devote a section to personnel to keep names and contact information about key personnel, graduate assistants, data collectors, technicians, and consultants. Update this contact information regularly as people move and positions change. Annual reports can go in another section/folder. If there have been changes for the IRB or the project must be reviewed, keep a section for just these reassurances. One section can be devoted to publications, abstracts, or news items about your study. For a multiyear grant, you may end up with a larger notebook or electronic file, or even two or three notebooks or electronic folders with subfolders. Binding your project together, both physically and virtually, in a retrievable form is essential to keeping track of your grant's history beyond the data you collect. It is more than a scrapbook of memorabilia; it is priceless when it comes time to write your final report to your grant funder.

* * *

ORDERING EQUIPMENT AND SUPPLIES

If you have planned well, you have prepared sufficient time to include procurement processes for equipment or supplies. This process differs from institution to institution. Know the guidelines for the purchase threshold for equipment purchases without external approval. These purchases can take time, and time consideration is particularly important when special instruments or devices must be made to order. Check with your institution's postaward accountant to see when you can start to spend funds. Some large institutions have mechanisms to order equipment when they receive a federal funding decision. Find out if you must make grant purchases through your institution's purchasing/receiving office. If so, clarify and supply information for sole-source items that cannot be replaced by less-expensive models for scientific reasons, and emphasize the urgency of expedient delivery to start your project. Also consider building on foundational equipment that is already in use at your institution. For example, if your research or educational project includes simulation equipment and there is already some equipment in place, buying from the same company often gains you discounts. Take advantage of loaner or rental equipment to train your personnel, and be innovative to avoid spinning your wheels.

* * *

WHEN CAN WE START?

Once your funds have been released to your institution, you will not be able to start your grant funded project until several things are in place. If yours is a federal grant, your office of research administration or grants and project office will make sure that you have met all required special project assurances, such as human subjects protection, protections for pregnant women, human fetuses and neonates involved in research, protections pertaining to biomedical and behavioral research involving prisoners as subjects, and additional protections for children involved as subjects in research. If you are using animals, you must produce clearances of your project from your institution's Institutional Animal Care and Use Committee. Any arrangements for ordering animals and housing them must also be cleared through your grants office. You need to complete any Conflict of Interest forms and resolve any outstanding IRB issues before you can begin your study. Finally, expect to talk with your purchasing office to negotiate and resolve any issues about the items being purchased for your study.

* * *

RECRUITING AND TRAINING PERSONNEL

As discussed in Chapter 4, you need to make plans for personnel well in advance of your funding notice. Once the grant is funded, you can begin to formalize these appointments, set up payroll arrangements, and in cases of salaried faculty or agency employees, set up new and realigned positions within the institution. Keeping in close communication with your accounting office during the grant application process makes this transition much easier. Many institutions require that you advertise positions for research staff with the human resources office that were not named as key personnel in your grant to comply with equal opportunity guidelines. Graduate research assistants may fall under a different category at your institution, so determine how these team members can be recruited. Take time and effort in picking your team. Consider recruiting students for research assistants. Graduate students often are able to find spin-off projects from engaging in studies. We have had success with employing undergraduate students for clinical studies, and with proper mentorship and supervision, they were reliable in collecting clinical data and enthusiastic about the work. Several of these students decided on graduate education, based on their experience with the study. Also, consider recruiting professional colleagues and nurses from clinical settings. Many would never consider embarking on a research study alone but are excellent data collectors or clinical experts. If you are posting an advertisement and interviewing persons you do not know, get professional references. Your project is a position of employment and requires reliable, ethical, and competent personnel. As discussed in Chapter 6, if your study involves community engagement with nonacademic partners and stakeholders, training about the project goals and processes should begin from the early formation of the partnership. Involving them early when they are expected to play an active part in the grant submission helps build their commitment as the grant is funded.

Training personnel often takes considerable time. If possible, plan a get-acquainted meeting of all your personnel well in advance of your study's start. Give each team member an abbreviated version of your research plan and explain each team member's role. Get everyone's schedule of availability, exchange contact phone numbers, and set up a training schedule. For studies that require an elaborate protocol, specialized instruments, and unusual data-collection schemes, have your team members practice the protocol on one another. Having someone serve as a surrogate subject may be helpful if you are training data collectors in dealing with a particular physical limitation or behavioral characteristic. Rehearsal of the protocol was most important in one study in which various stages of shivering were to be detected. We conducted inter-rater reliability tests on patients who shivered while recovering from anesthesia.

Here are some things to remember in the care and nurturing of a research team:

- **Build partnership/ownership among your team members.** Discuss study progress and acquaint them with the background and significance of the variables under study. Let them present parts of your orientation to the clinical or community sites.

- **Keep personnel happy and stimulated.** Grant teams are stimulated by learning more about the study. Celebrate holidays or special occasions with grant personnel with a cake or refreshments. Include them in seminar presentations, when appropriate.
- **Give periodic orientation and updates.** You need not feel compelled to prematurely share study findings with your team, but focus instead on the variables, their improvement in measurement, and spin-off ideas arising from their observations.
- **Find right roles and replacements.** Don't be imprisoned by the chores. Try constantly to work smarter and hold your team accountable for doing their designated roles within the study. If you are carrying out the work of others, stop and consider reassignments. You may find the person you have assigned to a project director role cannot direct others. If so, it is best to deal with this early; otherwise, you will be doing that person's job for them. If someone doesn't seem to fit in a research team role you first assigned, try something different. Let everyone experience success as much as possible, but do not neglect dealing with an absolute misfit in roles. Find the detail people on your team, and let them excel in record keeping and precision. Those that are better in social roles can be spokespersons or arrange meetings.
- **Clear understanding of data ownership**. Hard feelings arise after the fact if every team member thinks they can dip into the database and publish findings. Begin discussions early about who may do what with your study's data.
- **Clear authorship/presentation agreements.** As PI, you are responsible for the dissemination of research results, but you will likely generate findings that provide interesting observations for secondary data analysis. Make it clear from the beginning that any use of the data must be cleared with you before dissemination. At the same time, share the load and the opportunity with those who are contributors to the project's scientific work. Include coinvestigators in publication and presentations. If you have realistically included coinvestigators that contribute to your work, they deserve to share in the fruits of dissemination. On the other hand, consultants, research assistants, and persons employed to do various tasks on the study should not expect to be included in publications. Some publications now require that the percentage of time spent and the author's specific contribution be acknowledged at the time of submission. This practice discourages the PI from just listing the whole research team whether or not they contributed to the writing.

. . .

REMEMBER TO CARE FOR YOUR RESEARCH SITES

Cooperation from your clinical or community research site can either make or break a research study. Enlisting employees as coinvestigators or site coordinators in a hospital unit or clinical site can facilitate your access to subjects. Appointing clinical staff members as volunteer or official site coordinators gives them a feeling of ownership and may be a necessity for navigating an institution's internal IRB. Always include an orientation about your study for each shift so that they are aware what you are doing in the midst of their unit. If you have such valuable support from your research site, seek alternative rewards to show your gratitude. Sometimes, this can be in the form of coffee and bagels to show appreciation. You may also choose to make contributions to their unit library or leave behind equipment or teaching materials for them to keep. Always remember your research sites on holidays and special times. One way our project team chose to reward the clinical site over the December holidays was to bring a decorative bushel basket of apples (one for each shift). They loved the departure from candy and sweets over the holidays.

. . .

THINGS YOUR MOTHER MAY NEVER HAVE TOLD YOU

About Stewardship and Wise Spending

A grant is an endowment of trust. It is an investment in the future and a sign of faith that you can carry the project out. You are expected to be a thoughtful steward of this funding. Treat it as if you are the trusted treasurer of a highly respected association.

Who Keeps Books?

If you have a small grant with only a few items approved for purchase, keeping books is a snap. Your institution's accounting office informs you how you may purchase the items and how you should keep records and receipts because this becomes part of your report. Things become less clear-cut when you employ research assistants, give cash as remuneration to subjects, or deal with purchasing hourly services from a transcriptionist. You should keep an accounting of your spending, but you should engage services from your institution's accounting office to keep a paper trail that is available for audit. Each expense should be accounted for and clearly related to your budgeted award. There is some flexibility within categories for small changes in items, but always get clearance from your institution's postaward grant official for any changes you contemplate. Help dispel the myth that because you have a grant, all manner of things can now be charged to it. Along with your own care and stewardship, there are several other mechanisms that routinely audit and follow up on grant expenditures. Be parsimonious in your spending and pristine in your accounting and record keeping ("purer than Caesar's wife" comes to mind!). Expect questions to arise that you haven't thought of (How much does that lab rat cost? Who orders that lab rat? Where do we get pencils for those 100 people completing surveys today?). You can start your own collection of unanticipated questions. Try and keep a sense of humor. Some day they will make excellent anecdotes or will help in the making of a book on lessons learned.

Whose Money Is It?

Although you may be the PI of a grant, the funds may not be awarded to *you* personally. Federal grants are typically awarded to the institution in which the PI is employed. Your own institution may require that their office of research administration manage all grants, no matter how small. Although this may offend your sensibilities somewhat (who wrote this grant anyway?), the benefits outweigh any drawbacks. You get the scholarly credit and recognition, but the institution takes care of much of the big accounting chores, maintains your funds in a safe place, and keeps you in line with institutional assurances to the funding agency. In return, your institution gets indirect costs from large grants above and beyond those funding your research. A well-run office of research administration provides a repository for your funds and your information while making sure you maintain your fiscal agreements. If you change jobs and institutions during the period of the grant, be clear as to whether or not you can move the grant before you accept a new job and find out that the grant must remain behind.

•   •   •

CAVEAT TO THE SUCCESSFUL

Once the fatigue of waiting for your grant results is extinguished by the exhilaration of a grant award, beware of the feeling you may have of being "on a roll." You may feel like turning around and writing still another grant while you have the spirit. The feeling is similar to that of a new mother of twins who looks at the angelic babes on her lap and says, "Oh well, what's one more?" Unlike twins, you have a choice to put off taking on another grant until you have the first one well established. Your grant deserves undivided attention while you build your project team and nurture your project. Like twins, managing multiple studies takes more time. The more projects you are engaged in, the less time you have to write, think up new ideas, and relate to your project team. Stay focused; delay dashing off to write another grant until your present project is functioning well. Use your grant team to help you flesh out ideas for your next grant application.

New investigators often fall into a similar situation when they apply for and receive several small grants. The grantee may be caught up in the thrill of getting small grants without thinking ahead about the work involved with each. This may not create a problem if the grants were awarded to carry out different parts of the same study. Where the rub comes is when a grantee is successfully awarded several small grants to carry out two or three different studies at the same time. In most cases, these are local grants from organizations or foundations with little knowledge of how overcommitted the grantee is. The grantee likewise has not thought ahead beyond the wonderful prospect of "being funded." Small grants offer no salary support for the investigator so, along with a regular work schedule, the PI soon realizes that "just one more" means double the time commitment.

* * *

PROGRESS REPORTS ONCE THE FUNDING BEGINS

The same care that you took to write the grant must go into the submission of the progress reports. Although the form of progress reports may vary with funding institutions, you must attend to details carefully to ensure continuation or successful completion of your grant.

The cycle of progress reports depends on the funding agency. For a grant awarded for several years, such as a National Institutes of Health (NIH) research grant or a U.S. Department of Health and Human Services (USDHHS) Training grant, reports are annual *noncompeting* grant submissions. The acknowledgment of any changes that have occurred during the grant period and the progress made toward meeting the designated objectives/goals must be addressed in these reports. If a grant objective has not been met, then clearly state why. Ideally, you should be talking to your technical support person all along the grant's cycle, and the agency should already be aware of the problem. Even if they are aware, the problem and possible solution must be included in the report.

In the case of some grants, such as cooperative agreements from the Centers for Disease Control and Prevention, quarterly reports are required along with noncompeting grant renewals for each year of the grant. The guidelines for these reports must be followed to comply with the agency's regulations.

* * *

NONCOMPETING RENEWAL GRANTS

The funding cycle for a grant is 3 to 5 years for many federal grants. The second, third, and fourth years are referred to as *noncompeting grant renewal years*. This means that your project team or you, as the PI, are required to resubmit a streamlined *noncompeting continuation* grant application, including the grant's progress, budget usage or changes, and the proposed activities for the coming year. If Congress cuts federal funds to NIH or USDHHS drastically, grants could theoretically be cut as well. Because it was previously approved, your grant does not compete with new grant applications for funding. However, if the funding agency is dissatisfied with the grant's progress, they have the option to either decrease the funds or not renew the grant. Funded grants are rarely terminated unless there is a very good reason.

Renewal may be the time to request changes in budget lines. You generally need to make these requests in writing before funds can be moved from one budget line to another. But such budgetary changes certainly can be made at the time of noncompeting renewal. It is advisable to discuss the budgetary changes with your contact person at the agency before submitting the request as a part of your noncompeting renewal grant. Be as careful with these applications as you were with the first submission; they will be reviewed and scrutinized in most instances. Today's competitive world dictates an eye for detail in the renewal process.

Timelines for submissions of these reports can be just as sticky as the original grant application. Annual reports are generally required well in advance of a year. Sometimes an institution has an internal process for how these reports are sent. They may need to be reviewed by the department head, senior administrator, comptroller, or budget officer. Know these key people, the process, and their time frame for reviewing these reports.

* * *

PLANNING THE CONTINUATION

A successful grant not only accomplishes the project's goals and specific aims, but also generates meaningful questions that beg for answers. If your NIH research grant or training project has done that, you may wish to submit a *competing renewal* grant at the completion of your present grant if you have a compelling rationale to continue the same study with perhaps an enhanced population or approach. Not all levels of NIH funding allow competing renewals. Inquiries for all competing renewal applications should be directed to the NIH Program

Officer for the current grant. It is more likely that a new question or direction will cause you to write a new grant, perhaps moving from small grant funding (R03 or R15) to a large project (R01). Discuss your plans with your program office; write a concept paper or abstract of what you are considering. Address information your current funding has provided that moves you in this direction. Funding agencies look for their awards to generate new grant applications. Take advantage of the advice they offer.

• • •

LIFE AFTER GRANTS

There is really a life after grants! As a researcher/educator/practitioner, you must decide where you want your career to go after the grant is finished. It may be on to the next project or it may be to take a breather and really think about your next professional move. If you have not been successful at obtaining further funding, then perhaps this is a time to review other avenues for funding with a little different twist. For example, you might seek funds from Avon to examine the use of their skin care products in an adolescent population that has undergone chemotherapy with resultant dry skin. Or you might look at the use of complementary therapies in the treatment of women with endometriosis who are infertile. Although these two areas may not seem too out of line with current trends, they are not the usual mode of research for most nurses; the "twist" might give you a competitive edge. Another example is a nurse researcher with fibromyalgia who wants to compare time to diagnosis between health professionals and nonprofessionals. Again, this idea is not far from mainstream but has a new twist and may produce cost-effective results if one group is determined to obtain a diagnosis of fibromyalgia sooner than the other.

The time after a grant also affords you space to get the manuscripts and presentations written that seemed so elusive during the day-to-day administration of the grant. Presentations can be a joy when they come from your passion. Tell your story. Get people excited about you and your work. These presentations can also bring you into contact with other researchers or persons responsible for funding in your area. Remember that these presentations are selling your expertise and your work. A well-articulated presentation brings other opportunities for success. These opportunities may take your career in a slightly different direction than you had planned. Don't be afraid to go for the ride!

Don't underestimate the power of poster presentations. Many seasoned researchers or educators do not do posters. However, I find them very rewarding because novices ask many questions when you are standing by a poster; few will ask these questions in a large audience listening to an oral presentation. For the seasoned researcher, this is a time to be a good role model and help shape the career of a junior researcher. You can provide mentorship to another person. If you are the novice researcher or educator, a poster presentation is less intimidating than standing before the masses to orally present.

Take this time to renew your life. Too many times, nurses try to do it all. Let's face it: A grant and the work associated with it takes its toll on our lives and those of our family and friends. The time after a grant lets you renew your ties with the outside world. Some of you may laugh at that statement, but others know this to be true of either yourself or some of your colleagues. So take the time. Take that vacation. Go to that play you have been putting off for months. Renew your soul so you are ready for the next project.

CONCLUSION

Your grant award is a remarkable hallmark of your scholarship and one you can be justly proud of. However, the award is just the beginning of the work. Pick your team well; nurture and care for them, and they will reward you with good service. Take equal care of your research sites, and show your appreciation in tangible ways. Maintain the confidence and goodwill of your funding agency by submitting meticulously written, timely reports. When the project director or PI does not follow the guidelines or is habitually late on reports, funding agencies tend to question the management of the project. They are concerned about the team's commitment to the project for which they have supported with funds. Do not put yourself in that position. Put your best foot forward, and keep on track of the endless paper trail.

Finally, take time. Take care and maintain balance in your life. Life does go on and really is not grant dependent. Keep your sense of humor and laugh often! You will rarely find one's grant history carved on their tombstone.

RECOMMENDED READING FOR THE FUNDED GRANT WRITER

Cleary, M., Sayers, J., & Watson, R. (2016). Essentials of building a career in nursing research. *Nurse Researcher, 23*(60), 9–13. doi:10.7748/nr.2016.e1412

Eblen, M. K., Wagner, R. M., RoyChowdhury, D., Patel, K. C., & Pearshon, K. (2016). How criterion scores predict the overall impact score and funding outcomes for National Institutes of Health peer-reviewed applications. *PLOS ONE. Retrieved from* http://journals.plos.org/plosone/article?id=10.1371/journal.pone.0155060

Moxham, L. (2016). Nursing researchers forge careers in a highly competitive environment. *Nurse Researcher, 23*(6), 6–7. doi: 10.7748/nr.23.6.6.s2

11

Dissemination of Grant Findings

HARVESTING THE PRODUCTS OF RESEARCH

Nursing scholarship cannot advance without dissemination of findings from scientific research. Although the funding agency usually asks for a written report to learn of your study outcomes, your dissemination of scientific findings to a wider audience is even more important because it contributes to universal knowledge. The evidence base of nursing science grows with each contribution to the literature. In today's world of translational science, professional silos are fast disappearing. Your published study in a nursing journal may pique the interest of a scientist in a different discipline and even in a different country.

ADVANCING YOUR CAREER THROUGH DISSEMINATION

It is imperative for any grant recipient to complete a project by disseminating the outcomes of funded research. This final step in the grant process is a hallmark of an investigator's responsibility, capability, and contribution to scientific knowledge. Your scholarly career will be judged not only by your ability to obtain grants, but also by your ability to follow through to completion by dissemination to others. Acknowledge your collaborators' contribution through co-authorship and inclusion in other dissemination efforts. Scientific publications are the gold standard for dissemination because they are widely distributed and easily retrieved through literature databases such as MEDLINE, PubMed, or Cumulative Index to Nursing and Allied Health Literature (CINAHL). Publications of book chapters may give you entries in your curriculum vitae (CV), but are limited in distribution and nearly impossible for others to find from literature databases. One form of dissemination is an abstract/poster presentation. Podium or poster presentations can be ideal for dissemination of findings while awaiting journal publication if your selected scholarly journal allows it. However, podium or poster presentations should not take the place of a scientific publication. Sometimes, numerous abstract and poster presentations limit your time for writing manuscripts, so you must be more selective about choosing speaking engagements to allow more time for writing. For some researchers, the poster or abstract presentations act as springboards for manuscript submissions. These presentations also bring you into contact with others that may be doing similar research and offer great opportunities for networking. Others may procrastinate by doing presentations and move on to the next study without a written publication. Written dissemination of your data has the potential to contribute more to the scholarship of practice, teaching, and research resulting from a broader and more permanent avenue of dissemination. Remember the golden rule of research: If it is not disseminated, it is not considered done.

* * *

DEVELOPING A PLAN

Develop a dissemination plan for all aspects of your scholarship. As you begin to develop a program of research, opportunities exist for dissemination at various levels, including publication of literature reviews, theory development, pilot data, instrument development, primary and secondary research questions, serendipitous findings, and secondary analyses. A successful track record of dissemination can occur only if you make this aspect of your scholarship a priority. For most individuals, this means setting aside several hours a day or perhaps 1 day a week, depending on your schedule and writing style. Because writing can often take second place in a busy academic or clinical schedule, it is important to outline your publications and set timelines for submission to keep yourself on track.

As you begin your study, map the articles and spin-off publications you wish to write and set up a timeline. This is particularly important for community-engagement projects in which members may be unfamiliar with scientific publication. Engage your co-investigators and team members in presentations and publications appropriate to their contributions and interests. In our funded study on outcomes of fever in HIV, several spin-off projects emerged when doctoral students were involved. Some were able to participate in publishable literature reviews around variables under study. Others developed their own projects from secondary data.

When writing for publication, target your journal carefully based on the objectives you are trying to achieve. Know the audience of that journal. If the manuscript's goal is to reach clinicians in a timely manner, you may want to choose a clinical journal with a short publication schedule. If, however, data are not as time sensitive and the goal is to reach a broader audience, you may choose to submit your manuscript to a well-recognized, scholarly journal that has a larger subscription base but in which the timeline for publication following acceptance is longer.

The "journal impact factor" or various other bibliometrics may be important to consider when determining where to publish. Although publication numbers and the impact factor have traditionally been used to gauge a researcher's productivity for tenure and promotion, bibliometrics are also being used by funding agencies to determine which projects are worthier of funding and likely to give more return on investment (Argarwal et al., 2016).

Clinical intervention research often lends itself to a scholarly publication in a research journal and a practice-oriented description of the intervention in a clinical practice journal. In this case, the research from the scholarly journal can be cited and serves as a resource to the descriptive clinical article—but not a second research article. This approach makes it clear to a reader that you are not engaging in duplicate publication or "salami science," in which an author slices a research study into the thinnest possible slices to maximize the number of publications (Happell, 2016). The danger of "salami" slicing is that it inflates the results and gives the impression that more data exist to support a research question or hypothesis than actually do (Henly, 2014). Also, to ensure originality of publications, in dual publications, remember to be careful to avoid self-plagiarism by using new wording or quotation marks and referencing your work from the previous publication. If you plan to duplicate a table or figure from one of your previous publications, to avoid copyright infringement remember to get permission to republish the table or figure from the original publisher (Baggs, 2008).

In choosing journals, consider nursing and non-nursing, discipline-specific journals if the topic is of interest to professionals outside of nursing. Consider, too, that the reviewers may be researchers in your area or ones you have quoted, so make sure you are accurate. It is wise to see who is on the editorial board and review panel to see who might have published in your area. There is nothing worse than to have reviewers recognize that you have not acknowledged their work. Another word to the wise, following author guidelines is not optional. You must follow them. Once you have targeted a journal, see if there is a similar article on a different topic. Follow that format because, if they published that article, yours may have a greater chance of getting published. For example, my topic, "Transition from Hospital to Home for Mothers and Babies," might be similar to a hospital discharge and follow-up for an adult. If the latter article were published, then maybe mine might be too. In fact, it was. Be savvy when it comes to selecting and targeting a journal for disseminating your work.

• • •

PUBLISHING RESEARCH

Writing research findings may involve a new learning curve for a novice researcher. Even if you have published review or informative articles before, the process for publishing a research report is different. Unlike a dissertation, which may resemble a telephone book in size, the research article is usually no more than 16 pages and is crisp, concise, and free of extraneous verbiage. Your experience in writing a research grant is good preparation for writing research reports because it involves a stylized format and gets immediately to the point. Read examples of research reports from the journal in which you wish to publish. The journal's guide-to-the-author page or website should tell you if it has a recommended style or format for your submission.

Choose a journal that is likely to publish your methodology. Major nursing research journals, such as *Nursing Research, Research in Nursing and Health*, and *Western Journal of Nursing Research*, publish studies using both qualitative and quantitative approaches. Some have page limits that make it harder to include the rich narratives of qualitative studies. Others are highly supportive of this work, and a growing number of journals EW dedicated to or receptive of this methodology. A website sponsored by St. Louis University posts an extensive list of nursing and interdisciplinary journals accepting or focusing on qualitative research articles at www.slu.edu/organizations/qrc/QRjournals.html.

Although traditional journals available via hardcopy and/or electronic journal subscription have been the primary means for sharing research and scholarly findings, the availability for open-access publishing has dramatically changed the publication landscape. Open access publications provide free, unrestricted online access to digital scientific scholarly material by any user. These journals may request payment from the author to cover the costs of open access. Scholarly open-access journals retain many of the characteristics of traditional journals, including rigorous peer-review processes that maintain scholarly standards for publication. Unfortunately, the growth of open-access publishing has led to the growth and emergence of a number of online "predatory journals," which do not adhere to best practices and standards for scholarly publication (Oermann et al., 2016). To determine if the journal you have selected is a reputable journal and publisher, consult the Directory of Nursing Journals (nursingeditors. com/journals-directory). Also check the guidelines provided by the International Academy of Nursing Editors (INANE) to help evaluate the integrity of the nursing journal (Kearney and the INANE Predatory Publishing Practices Collaborative, 2015).

Some funding agencies have well-established policies requiring that publicly funded research be made accessible to readers for free with no subscription required. Most notably, the National Institutes of Health (NIH) Public Access Policy requires that all funded investigators submit an electronic version of their final, peer-reviewed publication to the NIH Manuscript Submission System on acceptance for publication and to the National Library of Medicine's PubMed Central no later than 12 months after the official date of publication.

Given the rapid explosion of information, many publishers have begun to assign digital object identifiers (DOIs). DOIs provide a lasting embedded hyperlink to make the journal publication quick and easy to locate and track (Schwarz, 2014).

Examine samples of articles from a variety of journals and shop around before you choose where you submit your article. Carefully evaluate the journal's characteristics and the publisher's business practices before selecting a journal for publication. Take the time to examine the mission and format of the journal to see if it provides the best audience for the report you intend to publish. Choosing between a research and a practice journal may require a decision about which would meet both the professional and the clinical interests of the reader. Fortunately, many clinical and practice journals have incorporated research reports into their publications.

* * *

WHAT DO EDITORS WANT?

Aspiring authors should understand that editors *do* want to publish articles, even though the review process is sometimes harsh. In truth, editors are seeking well-written articles and actively trying to tell us what they want. Recent nursing research editorials have provided tips and guidelines to help authors write more competitive manuscripts. One editor surveyed other journal editors to see what they wanted, what mistakes authors made, and what delighted the editors (Froman, 2008a, 2008b, 2011). In some cases, editors expressed joy, even ecstasy, over a well-written article. Some editors express similar emotions over an author who followed submission directions. The tips are easy to understand and can help direct you to avoid jargon, use of pseudosophisticated words, and complicated sentences. Headaches come from authors who disregard the journal's format or mission, length restrictions, and required materials. Don't be put off by requests to revise. As one editor described it, "rigorous peer review is a gift to the journal and the author" (Kearney, 2016). Most articles require some revision, so if you are given the opportunity to clarify and tighten your manuscript, you have been given the gift of revision (Bearinger, Taliaferro, & Given, 2010). Try to bear in mind that the rigorous review is aimed at reporting accurate, well-conducted studies with appropriate measurements, analyses, and interpretation.

When faulty research is published, it misleads research consumers. Therefore, reviewers take their task seriously. They must overlook reports that are exciting, catchy, or highly readable and point out problems in research that was poorly designed with findings not justified by the evidence.

• • •

EXPECT TO COMPETE

Getting published is not a shoo-in just because your grant was funded. Like grantsmanship, you must expect to compete. Get help if writing the manuscript seems an onerous task. Writing of any kind gets easier the more you practice it. Engage help from your statistical consultant before writing quantitative findings. If someone on your grant team shines in writing, let that person help you organize the research report. Have plenty of review from colleagues and experts before submission. To increase your manuscript acceptance rate, you may want to consider setting up a process for scientific review of your manuscripts before submission. Select the reviewers based on the type of feedback you are seeking for your manuscript (e.g., copy editing, design and methods, or clinical implications). Do not be discouraged or defeated by a rejected manuscript. Although rejection by a journal editor can be difficult, remember that it was the article, not *you*, that was being rejected. Articles can be reworked. Take the comments provided and use them to improve the manuscript. Ultimately, you may choose to resubmit to the same journal or even a different journal after careful evaluation of the journal's target audience. Occasionally, you may find that the same reviewer receives your manuscript to review when you submit it to a different journal. This often happens when you write in a specialized area. For this reason, take the time and effort to make any recommended changes and rethink areas that received negative comments. When submitting a manuscript, have both a primary and a secondary journal in mind to facilitate the resubmission process.

Finally, you need to evaluate your dissemination plan periodically and adjust it as necessary. This evaluation should include your publication submission-to-acceptance ratio. You might find that you need to reorganize your scholarship priorities to increase your publication output. Perhaps you need to develop more realistic goals and timelines for publications.

CONCLUSION

Dissemination of your findings is exciting. Few ego boosts equal seeing your name in print on a widely disseminated article. Publication allows you to share your information and build a niche for yourself as you build a professional career. Writing and disseminating through presentations become your legacy to the profession and to your family. Like any scholarly endeavor, the more you practice, the greater the ease and sophistication of your product. The struggle may be real, but the opportunities abound for you to disseminate your work.

REFERENCES

Argarwal, A., Durairajanayagam, D., Tatagari, S., Esteves, S. C., Harlev, A., Henkel, R., ... Bashiri, A. (2016). Bibliometrics: Tracking research impact by selecting the appropriate metrics. *Asian Journal of Andrology*, *18*(2), 296–309. doi:10.4103/1008-682X.171582

Baggs, J. G. (2008). Issues and rules for authors concerning authorship versus acknowledgements, dual publication, self-plagiarism, and salami publishing. *Research in Nursing & Health*, *31*(1), 295–297. doi:10.1002/nur.20280

Bearinger, L. H., Taliaferro, L., & Given, B. (2010). When R & R is not rest & recovery but revise & resubmit. *Research in Nursing & Health*, *33*(5), 381–385. doi:10.1002/nur.20398

Froman, R. D. (2008a). Hitting the bull's eye rather than shooting yourself between the eyes. *Research in Nursing & Health*, *31*(5), 399–401. doi:10.1002/nur.20296

Froman, R. D. (2008b). Polishing your shot at the bull's eye: The "please do" list. *Research in Nursing & Health*, 31(6), 541–542. doi:10.1002/nur.20301

Froman, R. D. (2011). Format, style, and precision. *Research in Nursing & Health*, *34*(1), 1–3. doi:10.1002/nur.20414

Happell, B. (2016). Salami: By the slice or swallowed whole? *Applied Nursing Research*, *30*, 29–31. doi:10.1016/j.apnr.2015.08.011

Henly, S. J. (2014). Duplicate publications and salami reports: Corruption of the scientific record. *Nursing Research*, *63*(1), 1–2. doi:10.1097/NNR.0000000000000015

Kearney, M. H. (2016). Rigorous peer review is worth the effort. *Research in Nursing & health*, *39*(6), 393–395. doi:10.1002/nur.21771

Kearney, M. H., & The INANE Predatory Publishing Practices Collaborative. (2015). Predatory publishing: What authors need to know. *Research in Nursing & Health*, *38*(1), 1–3. doi:10.1002/nur.21640

Oermann, M. H., Conklin, J. L., Nicoll, L. H., Chinn, P., Ashton, K. S., Idie, A. H., ... Budinger, S. C. (2016). Study of predatory open access nursing journals. *Journal of Nursing Scholarship*, *48*(6), 624–632. doi:10.1111/jnu.12248

Schwarz, L. m. (2014). DOI? Why? How to questions and answers. *CIN: Computers, Informatics, Nursing*, 32(2), 51–53. doi:10.1097/CIN.0000000000000047

U.S. Department of Health and Human Services. (2017). NIH public access policy details. Retrieved from https://publicaccess.nih.gov/policy.htm

Glossary

Academic Research Enhancement Award (R-15): NIH mechanism used to support small research projects conducted by faculty in educational institutions that have not been major participants in NIH programs.

Application identification number: Unique number assigned to a submitted NIH application that identifies (in this order): Type of application (e.g., 1 = new, 2 = competing continuation), activity code (e.g., R01), serial number assigned by the Center for Scientific Review (e.g., 143723), suffix showing the support year for the grant (e.g., the first year of a grant would be 01), and other information identifying a supplement (e.g., S1), amendment (e.g., A1), or other modifying data. A sample application identification number would be 1 R01 A1 143723 01 A1 S1.

Career Development Awards (K Awards): NIH series of grant awards to support PhDs and clinicians wishing to develop careers in biomedical research. The level of award (K1 through K99) depends on the type and level of training, research, or mentorship.

Clinical and Translational Science Awards (CTSA): NIH initiative to accelerate research.

Collaborative Institutional Training Initiative (CITI): Online training to prepare a researcher for human subjects' protection and to promote scientific integrity.

Computer Retrieval of Information on Scientific Projects (CRISP): Biomedical database system containing information on research projects and programs supported by the U.S. Department of Health and Human Services and specifically the U.S. Public Health Service. Searchable by name, institution, funding institute, date, and topic, the CRISP website (https://www.nlm.nih.gov/research/umls/sourcereleasedocs/current/CSP) is a good place to search for scientific concepts, emerging trends, and techniques or to identify specific projects and/or investigators.

Contract: Award that establishes a binding legal procurement relationship between the NIH and an award recipient, obligating the latter to provide a product or service defined in detail by the NIH and binding the institute to pay for it.

Cooperative agreement: Form of grant that usually requires the grantee and grantor to work together after the funding begins to formulate research protocols.

Data monitoring and safety: Plan required by the NIH for clinical trials but also applied to other research. It refers to the responsibility of the researcher-principal investigator (PI) to identify how data, human subjects' information, and safety of the subjects are provided. The plan must include what an adverse event is and how it is identified, handled, and reported.

Direct costs: Expenses, such as salaries, equipment specifically designated for the project, and other monies that go to support the project.

Evidence-based practice: Use of scientific data, clinical expertise, and patient preferences that is synthesized to support clinical interventions.

Facilities and administrative costs (F&A): Costs that are budgeted on grants for several common or joint objectives and cannot be specifically identified with a particular project or program. Commonly known as *indirect costs.*

Gantt chart: A visual use of bar graphs to depict timelines for various aspects of a project.

***Healthy People 2020* objectives:** Current decade-specific initiatives to improve the U.S. health outcomes.

***Healthy People 2030* objectives:** Planning now underway for science-based, 10 year national objectives to improve health of all Americans.

Indirect costs: Expenses or overhead that it takes to run a grant: benefits packages, cost of utilities, phone cost, legal services for contracts, and other hidden costs that are part of the bricks and mortar of conducting daily business in any institution. Also known as *facilities and administrative costs (F&A).*

Interprofessional Education Collaborative (IPEC): Work aimed at improving population health outcomes through teamwork.

Institutional review board (IRB): Review panel made up of professionals and at least one or two laypersons that examines the ethics, safety, and scientific merit of the research only in relationship to participant rights. Human subjects' protection is the aim of this panel, which resides in the hospital where the research, educational, or special project is conducted; an academic institution; or both. A central IRB may be used as the single, IRB of record for multi-center clinical trials.

National Database for Nursing Quality Indicators (NDNQI): Initiative to test nursing-sensitive quality indicators to improve quality of care.

NIH Clinical Trial Planning Grant (R34): Grant that supports peer review of the foundation of a clinical trial and the development of a clinical trial intervention.

NIH Exploratory/Developmental Research Grant Award (R21): Development of research in a new area. May include pilot and feasibility studies.

NIH High-Priority, Short-Term Project Award (R56): Grants for new or competing renewal applications whose priority funding may not have been within the "awarded" range.

NIH Program Project/Center Grants (P Series): Grants aimed at the development of multipronged projects that fall under one umbrella constituting a center. These may be exploratory grants. The P series includes P01, P20, P30, and P50.

NIH Research Project Grant Program (R01): Research grants to support original health-related research in a very specific area supported by the researcher's area of expertise.

NIH Research Projects (R25): Grants that support educational projects, including program coordination and evaluation.

NIH Roadmap: Plan by NIH to guide research in the 21st century.

NIH Small Grant Program (R03): Two-year funding mechanism for pilot or feasibility studies, secondary analysis of existing data, development of new technology, or collection of preliminary data.

NIH Support for Conferences and Scientific Meetings (R13 and U13): Support for high-level, quality meetings aligned with NIH's roadmap.

National Research Service Awards (NRSA): Grants to support collaborative research opportunities and predoctoral and postdoctoral fellowships. They include F05, F30, F31, F32, F33, and F99/K00.

Noncompeting continuation: Continued support for an NIH-funded grant. Progress reports for continued support do not undergo peer review but are administratively reviewed by the institute/center and receive an award based on prior award commitments. Also known as *Type 5*.

Noncompeting grant: Ongoing grant whose award is contingent on the completion of a progress report as the condition for the release of money for the following year. Award is predicted on solid evidence that the grant is doing what it set out to do.

Patient-Centered Outcomes Research Institute (PCORI): Research center aimed at helping patients, families, and clinicians address health problems with reliable information and clinical effectiveness to improve clinical decision making.

Power analysis: Method by which a sample size is calculated to achieve significance. This analysis considers the level of significance of the variable of interest, the effect size desired, and finally the number of subjects it will take to achieve significant results.

Qualitative research: method of research that looks at the subjective worldview. The concern is to describe "what is" rather than predict why an event occurred.

Quantitative research: Research method interested in quantifying or counting responses. This type of research answers questions of relationships, probability, causality, and predictability. Objective, verifiable data are of interest.

Randomized controlled trial (RCT): "Gold standard" of research because there is a control group compared with at least one other group that receives an intervention.

Request for applications (RFA): Call for grantees to apply for research or educational funds. These calls designate the objectives for the grant monies, the type of grant accepted for review, and the cycle for the grant from application to the funding announcement.

Request for proposals (RFP): Same as a Request for Applications but on a broad range of research priorities versus a specific designated priority area. Also called *call for grant applications*.

Scientific review administrator (SRA): NIH scientist-administrator who presides over a scientific review group, coordinates the meeting, and reports the review of each application assigned to it. The SRA serves as an intermediary between the applicant and reviewers and prepares summary statements for all applications reviewed.

Small Business Innovation Research (SBIR) and Small Business Technology Transfer (STTR) Grants: NIH-sponsored programs that support projects to establish the technical merit and feasibility of research and development ideas leading to commercial products or services.

Special Projects of Regional and National Significance (SPRANS): Grant funds to support projects that support a regional or national healthcare need.

Summary statements: Combined reviewers' written comments and the Scientific Review Administrator's summary of the review panel's discussion during the study section meeting. It includes the recommendations of the study section, a recommended budget, and administrative notes of special considerations.

Sustainable Development Goals (SDGs): Objectives set by the United Nations to improve health outcomes globally by addressing education, poverty, hunger, and climate change.

Systematic or integrated reviews: Reviews of literature, usually of randomized clinical controlled trials that represent the state of the science on a specific topic. Databases on the Internet house these reviews that provide evidence to support a grant area or an intervention.

Web Resources

This resource section is not meant to be comprehensive but to give the reader an idea of possible grant sources and how to search for grants, write grants, do statistical analyses, and disseminate findings.

Grant Funding Sources (corporations, foundations, governmental, nongovernmental, professional organizations)

Agency for Healthcare Research and Quality (AHRQ): http://www.ahrq.gov/funding/policies/foaguidance/index.html
Information and guidance about grants—how to apply, funding priorities, types of grants available.

American Nurses Foundation (ANF): http://www.anfonline.org/nursingresearchgrant
Call for applications, list of available grants, online application, and past funded grants.

American Organization of Nurse Executives (AONE) Foundation: http://www.aone.org
Available small grants.

American Public Health Association (APHA): https://www.apha.org/policies-and-advocacy/public-health-policy-statements/policy-database/2014/07/15/15/58/federal-grants-and-public-health
Focus on public health issues, policy initiatives.

Arnold P. Gold Foundation: http://www.gold-foundation.org/programs-old/
   apply-for-a-grant
Most interested in humanistic health.

Bill and Melinda Gates Foundation: http://www.gatesfoundation.org/How-We-Work/
   General-Information/Grant-Opportunities
Opportunities for grants that impact health globally.

Canadian Institutes of Health Research (CIHR): http://www.cihr-irsc.gc.ca/e/193
   .html
Multiple areas of research funding.

Centers for Disease Control and Prevention (CDC): https://www.cdc.gov/grants/
   index.html
Grant opportunities along with information about how to apply, federal regulations and policies, and funding profiles. These grants are cooperative
   agreements that are shaped with input from the CDC and address US and
   global initiatives.

Computer Retrieval of Information on Scientific Projects (CRISP): https://www
   .nlm.nih.gov/research/umls/sourcereleasedocs/current/CSP
Biomedical database system containing information on research projects funded
   by the U.S. Public Health Service.

Gordon and Betty Moore Foundation: https://www.moore.org/grants
Grants offered in a wide variety of areas.

Health Resources & Services Administration (HRSA): https://www.hrsa.gov/grants/
   apply
Many grant opportunities, especially for educational programs and a quick guide
   for grant applications.

Interact for Health (formerly Health Foundation of Greater Cincinnati): https://www
   .interactforhealth.org/our-history
Resource for grants in the Ohio region.

Interprofessional Education Collaborative (IPEC): https://www.ipecollaborative
   .org/funding-opportunities.html
Grants in conjunction with other organizations such as Robert Wood Johnson
   Foundation, Gordon and Betty Moore Foundation, John A. Hartford
   Foundation, and Josiah Macy, Jr. Foundation. Focus on interprofessional
   educational projects.

John A. Hartford Foundation: http://www.johnahartford.org/grants-strategy
Focus on aging and issues around elder care.

Josiah Macy Jr. Foundation: http://macyfoundation.org/apply
Interested in education and training, especially interprofessional projects.

March of Dimes Birth Defects Foundation: http://www.marchofdimes.org/research/
research-grants.aspx
Research grants and past funded projects.

National Institutes of Health (NIH): https://grants.nih.gov/funding/index.htm
Grant opportunities along with research training opportunities.

National Science Foundation: https://www.nsf.gov
Focus on science and engineering.

Patient-Centered Outcomes Research Institute (PCORI): http://www.pcori.org/
funding-opportunities
All open funding opportunities as well as research dissemination of comparative
effectiveness research and other PCORI-funded studies.

Robert Wood Johnson Foundation: http://www.rwjf.org
Focus on creating a culture of health.

Sigma Theta Tau International (STTI): https://www.nursingsociety.org
Research awards and a place for dissemination of research through conference
presentations.

*Small Business Innovation Research (SBIR) and Small Business Technology Transfer
(STTR)*: https://sbir.nih.gov
Grants to support business start-ups and creation of technology.

Substance Abuse and Mental Health Services Administration (SAMHSA): https://
www.samhsa.gov/grants
Grants focused on substance abuse and mental health support programs.

Dissemination

American Organization of Nurse Executives (AONE): http://www.aone.org
Supports dissemination of research/educational projects at annual conferences.

American Psychological Association (APA): http://www.apa.org/research/responsible/
publication
Outlines author's responsibility in disseminating research findings.

Council for the Advancement of Nursing Science (CANS): http://www
.nursingscience.org/about/council-history
Supports research awards, research networking opportunities, and dissemination
of work.

Eastern Nursing Research Society (ENRS): http://www.enrs-go.org
Offers research awards and a place for dissemination of research through conference presentations.

Midwest Nursing Research Society (MNRS): https://www.mnrs.org/
mnrs%E2%80%93developing-new-generations-nurse-scientists
Offers research awards, grant opportunities, and a place for dissemination of research through conference presentations.

Southern Nursing Research Society (SNRS): https://www.snrs.org
Offers research awards, grant opportunities, and a place for dissemination of research through conference presentations.

Western Institute of Nursing (WIN): https://www.winursing.org
Offers research awards, grant opportunities, and a place for dissemination of research through conference presentations.

Grant Writing Tools

American Psychological Association (APA): http://www.apa.org/research/responsible/
publication
Assistance in the writing and dissemination of research finding.

Cochrane Library—Cochrane Database of Systematic Reviews (CDSR): http://www
.cochranelibrary.com/cochrane-database-of-systematic-reviews
Good source for systematic reviews and protocols to support grant writing literature review sections.

Collaborative Institutional Training Initiative (CITI): https://www.citiprogram.org
One form of research training to prepare for an IRB submission. Some institutions require NIH research/ethical training.

Dun & Bradstreet Data Universal Numbering System (D-U-N-S): http://www.dnb
.com/duns-number.html
Research submitted to the U.S. government requires the principal investigator/
project director to have a D-U-N-S number.

Electronic Research Administration (eRA) Commons: https://public.era.nih.gov/
commons
Central hub for NIH grant activities.

Foundation Center: http://foundationcenter.org/products/foundation-grants-to
-individuals-online
Searchable foundation grants database available by subscription.

Grants.gov: https://www.grants.gov

Great resources for research training and funding for research and educational projects.

Grants Resource Center—American Association of State Colleges and Universities (AASCU): http://www.aascu.org/GRC
Resource with a searchable grants database. Alerts can be sent through email as grants become available in a researcher's area of interest.

Grant Siren: http://www.grantwriters.net
Grant writing group available to assist those seeking funding.

Healthy People 2020: https://www.healthypeople.gov
Lists of the progress to date since Healthy People 2020 started. Some grants require that the researcher include information about the U.S. Health Indicators and refer to the blueprint from this project. The agency works in partnership with the American Public Health Association (APHA) and attempts to address health disparities.

Healthy People 2030: https://www.healthypeople.gov/2020/About-Healthy-People/Development-Healthy-People-2030
On development of the next decade of science-based, 10-year national objectives to improve health of all Americans. The site includes: Draft of framework, Public comment, Advisory Committee, and scheduled Committee meetings. The Advisory meeting makes recommendations to the Secretary of Health and Human Services regarding the Healthy People 2030 initiative.

Institutional Review Board (IRB): http://www.american.edu/irb/index.cfm
One example of IRB guidelines. Consult your own institution's information. This one is from the American University of Washington, DC.

Joanna Briggs Institute (JBI): http://joannabriggs.org
Good source for critical appraisals of literature, as well as training on how to conduct systematic reviews.

National Institutes of Health (NIH): https://nexus.od.nih.gov/all/2017/05/19/new-tutorials-on-preparing-and-submitting-your-nih-grant-application/?utm_source=nexus&utm_medium=email&utm_content=nihupdate&utm_campaign=may17
New tutorials on preparing and submitting NIH grant applications. Video goes through the process.

National Institutes of Health (NIH): https://grants.nih.gov/grants/about_grants.htm
Overview of the grant process.

National Institutes of Health (NIH): https://grants.nih.gov/grants/how-to-apply
-application-guide/video/prepare-to-apply/index.htm
Four-part series on YouTube to describe how to apply for NIH grants.

New Jersey Big Data Alliance: http://njbda.weebly.com
Training available to address state workforce issues using big data and public
access to Big Data Resources.

NVivo: http://www.qsrinternational.com/nvivo-product
One example of a qualitative analysis software package.

SAS: https://www.sas.com/en_us/solutions/analytics.html?keyword=sta
tistical%252520software&matchtype=p&publisher=google&gclid=
CMG_ufWLw9QCFRNYDQodPQoKMA
Statistical software used mainly in the social sciences.

*SMARTS™ funding alerts (a service of InfoEd Global's SPIN™ funding opportuni-
ties)*: http://infoedglobal.com
Grants database available to researchers and those in higher education. Grant
alerts can be set up to be delivered via email on a regular basis.

SMOG (Simple Measure of Gobbledygook) Readability Formula: http://www
.readabilityformulas.com/smog-readability-formula.php
Tool that helps determine the reading level of forms such as informed consents.

SPSS Software—IBM Analytics: https://www.ibm.com/analytics/us/en/technology/
spss
One example of a statistical analysis package available for purchase.

Sustainable Development Goals (SDGs): http://www.un.org/sustainabledevelopment/
sustainable-development-goals
Some global grants refer to the Millennium Development Goals (MDGs), http://
www.who.int/topics/millennium_development_goals/en, that were started
by the United Nations to address global morbidity and mortality. These led
to the creation of the SDGs that consist of 17 goals to address world issues,
several of which address health.

Vermont Oxford Network: https://public.vtoxford.org
Neonatal-focused database available through membership.

Index

Printed in the United States
By Bookmasters